30, 31
46, 47, 48, 49
51, 96-97
175

Chemical Dependency and Intimacy Dysfunction

Chemical Dependency and Intimacy Dysfunction

Eli Coleman, PhD
Editor

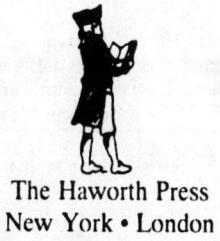

The Haworth Press
New York • London

Chemical Dependency and Intimacy Dysfunction has also been published as *Journal of Chemical Dependency Treatment*, Volume 1, Number 1 1987.

© 1988 by The Haworth Press, Inc. All rights reserved. No part of this work may be reproduced or utilized in any form or by any means, electronic or mechanical, including photocopying, microfilm and recording, or by any information storage and retrieval system, without permission in writing from the publisher. Printed in the United States of America.

The Haworth Press, Inc., 12 West 32 Street, New York, NY 10001
EUROSPAN/Haworth, 3 Henrietta Street, London WC2E 8LU England

Library of Congress Cataloging-in-Publication Data

Chemical dependency and intimacy dysfunction.

   "Has also been published as Journal of chemical dependency treatment, volume 1, number 1, fall/winter 1987" – T.p. verso.
   Includes bibliographies.
   1. Substance abuse – Patients – Sexual Behavior. 2. Psychosexual disorders. 3. Substance abuse – Patients – Family relationships. 4. Substance abuse – Patients – Mental Health. I. Coleman, Eli. [DNLM: 1. Sex Behavior – drug effects. 2. Sex Disorders – chemically induced. 3. Substance Dependence – complications. WM 270 C515]
RC564.C476   1987   616.85'83   87-26173
ISBN 0-86656-640-6
ISBN 0-86656-826-3 (pbk.)

Dedication

To Timothy and the rest of my "family"

Chemical Dependency and Intimacy Dysfunction

CONTENTS

Foreword *David E. Smith, MD*	1
Preface *Eli Coleman, PhD*	3
Introduction *Eli Coleman, PhD*	7
Chemical Dependency and Intimacy Dysfunction: Inextricably Bound *Eli Coleman, PhD*	13
Definitions	14
The Correlations and Relationships of Intimacy Dysfunction and Chemical Abuse and Dependency	17
What Do These Correlations Mean?	20
Conclusion	22
Child Physical and Sexual Abuse Among Chemically Dependent Individuals *Eli Coleman, PhD*	27
Child Physical Abuse and Neglect	27
Fetal Alcohol Syndrome	29
Sexual Abuse	29
Shame	31
Boundary Inadequacy	32
Perpetrators of Incest	33
Conclusion Regarding Sex Offenders	36
Conclusion	36

Marital and Relationship Problems Among Chemically Dependent and Codependent Relationships   **39**
Eli Coleman, PhD

Codependency	40
Sexual Identity Conflicts	42
Violence in Relationships	46
Confusion of Roles in the Relationship	48
Communication Difficulties	49
Intimacy and Sexual Attitudes and Values	50
Sexual Dysfunction	52
Conclusion Regarding Marital-Relationship Difficulties	55

Shame, Intimacy, and Sexuality   **61**
Jeffrey A. Brown, MSE

Formation of Shame	62
Formation of Shame-Related Intimacy Dysfunction	63
Formation of Sexual Shame	65
Intimacy and Shame in Adulthood	68
Sexual Shame in Adulthood	69
Overview of Intervention/Treatment	70
A Treatment Model	72

Assessment of Boundary Inadequacy in Chemically Dependent Individuals and Families   **75**
Philip Colgan, MA

Boundary Inadequacy	76
Dependence and Caring	77
Interdependence and Individual Differences	78
Independence and Personal Power	79
The Assessment	80
Psychological Boundary Issues	81
Physical Boundary Issues	83
Assessment: The Role of the Clinician	84
Summary	88

Women, Sexuality and the Process of Recovery   **91**
Susan Schaefer, MA
Sue Evans, MA

Sexual Dissatisfaction/Dysfunction	92
Sex Role Conflicts	94

Intimacy and Interpersonal Relationships	94
Sexual Orientation	96
Sexual Abuse/Incest	96
Factors Impacting the Relationship Between Women's Sexuality and Recovery	97
Physical Correlates	100
Shame	106
Guilt	108
Depression	108
Grief	109
Spiritual Aspects	110
Addendum I	113

Sexual Orientation Concerns Among Chemically Dependent Individuals — 121
        Susan Schaefer, MA
        Sue Evans, MA
        Eli Coleman, PhD

Socio-Political Influences Producing Higher Rates of Alcohol Abuse	125
Special Treatment Considerations	127
Sexual Orientation Issues in Recovery	130
Recommendations	136

Incest and Chemically Dependent Women: Treatment Implications — 141
        Sue Evans, MA
        Susan Schaefer, MA

The Role of Socialization	144
Incest as an Intergenerational Phenomenon	146
Boundary Formation	147
Definitions of Incest	150
Psychological Precursors of Incest	157
Incest Assessment	160
I. Behavioral Cues for the Diagnosis of Incest	160
II. Psychological Cues for the Diagnosis of Incest	162
III. Covert Familial Cues: Did Anyone in Your Family Ever . . .	163
Recommendations	164
Suggestions for Working with Clients	165

Identifying the Male Chemically Dependent Sex Offender and a Description of Treatment Methods   **175**
Margretta Dwyer, RSM, MA

Patterns of a Sex Offender	176
Demographics	177
Percentage Who Are Chemically Dependent	178
Treatment Issues	178
Which Comes First	179
Assessment	179
Key Elements of a Treatment Program	180
Treatment Modalities	182
Conclusion	186

Sexual Compulsivity: Definition, Etiology, and Treatment Considerations   **189**
Eli Coleman, PhD

Definition	190
Treatment Approaches	192
The Debate Over Terminology	194
Etiology	196
Relationship to Chemical Dependency	198
Conclusion and Summary	202

Treatment of Dependency Disorders in Men: Toward a Balance of Identity and Intimacy   **205**
Philip Colgan, MA

The Problem: Dependency Disorders	205
Identity Disorders	206
Intimacy Dysfunction	207
Etiology	210
Intimacy Dysfunction: The Family	210
Development of Patterns of Over-Separation and Over-Attachment	211
Relationships Outside the Family: Further Development of Over-Attachment and Over-Separation Patterns	213
Patterns of Dependency Disorders in Adult Relationships	215
The Cycle of Over-Separation	216
The Cycle of Over-Attachment	218
Treatment Considerations	220

Identity Development	222
Intimacy	223
Identity and Intimacy	224
Summary	226

Treating Intimacy Dysfunctions in Dyadic Relationships Among Chemically Dependent and Codependent Clients   229
Sondra Smalley, MA
Eli Coleman, PhD

Overt and Covert Forms of Codependency	231
The Underlying Beliefs of Codependency	232
Characteristics of Codependency	233
Is This Pattern a Disease or a Pattern?	233
Treatment Strategies	234
Stage One—Focusing on Identity	235
Stage Two—Focusing on Interaction with Others	238
Stage Three—Focusing on the Dyadic Relationship	240
Conclusion	241

Toward a Healthy Sexual Lifestyle Post Chemical Dependency Treatment   245
Sandra L. Nohre, MA

Description of the Problems	246
Sexuality Issues	246
Definition of Sexuality	247
Role of Sex Therapy	249
Steps Toward a Healthy Sexual Lifestyle	250
Intimacy and Trust	256
Intimacy and Sex	257
Case Illustration	257
Conclusion	259

Intimacy, Aging and Chemical Dependency   261
John Brantner, PhD

Intimacy and Aging	263
Intimacy and Alcohol	265
Treatment	266

Chemical Dependency and Intimacy Dysfunction

ABOUT THE EDITOR

Eli Coleman, PhD, is Associate Professor and the Associate Director at the Program in Human Sexuality of the Department of Family Practice and Community Health, Medical School, University of Minnesota. Dr. Coleman is a Licensed Consulting Psychologist and a certified sex therapist. Dr. Coleman is internationally recognized as an expert on sexuality, especially in the areas of alcoholism and sexuality, homosexuality, and sexual dysfunction. He has contributed more than a dozen chapters to textbooks in the area of sexuality. His other credits include numerous articles for scholarly and scientific journals, including the *American Behavioral Scientist*, the *Journal of Counseling and Development* (formerly the *Personnel and Guidance Journal*), and the *Journal of Homosexuality*. He is also on the Editorial Board of the *Journal of Homosexuality* and is the Special Editor of an upcoming issue of the Journal on new psychotherapeutic approaches. He is also editing a special issue of the *Family Practice Research Journal* devoted to human sexuality. Finally, Haworth Press has invited him to be the Editor of a new journal entitled *The Journal of Psychology and Human Sexuality*.

Dr. Coleman has been the coordinator of a national training program in Chemical Dependency and Family Intimacy. This training program began in 1979 and hundreds of professionals from around the country have been trained.

The other authors have been members of the faculty of this training program. They are accomplished clinicians who have the theoretical and academic background needed to communicate their skills. They offer unique theories and techniques as well as a recognition of the contributions others have made to understanding and treating these problems.

Foreword

Eli Coleman and his associates are one of the world's leading groups in the study of chemical dependence and human sexuality. This publication represents the key issues in their multidisciplinary approach to the study of this complicated area.

Unfortunately, the fields of chemical dependence and human sexuality have relatively little cross-fertilization to the detriment of both fields. This publication can help to bridge this gap between chemical dependency and human sexuality, improving the level of understanding and the quality of care in both areas.

Failure to deal with social-sexual issues may impair the progress of recovery in a chemically dependent individual and his or her family. Failure to deal with sexual compulsivity in intravenous drug abusers may seriously impair our ability to deal with Acquired Immunodeficiency Syndrome (AIDS), which is associated with both chemical dependence and frequent, anonymous sex. Failure to deal with chemical dependence may render daily therapy ineffective in the treatment of sex offenders. Failure to be sensitive to women or sexual minority issues may render chemical dependence treatment in these areas ineffective.

The list goes on and on, and the issues are clearly important. Eli Coleman and associates, through their pioneering work have helped to address the need for professionals in the fields of chemical dependence and human sexuality to understand the importance of each other's work, and the need for further integration of these two fields.

I applaud the efforts of these fine researchers and professionals, and hope that this publication can serve the important role of bridging these two areas in the helping professions.

David E. Smith, MD
Founder and Medical Director
Haight-Ashbury Free Medical Clinics
Co-Editor, Sexological Aspects of Substance Use and Abuse
Journal of Psychoactive Drugs, *Volume 14, No 1-2*

Preface

In 1978, I joined the faculty and staff of the Program in Human Sexuality after receiving my doctorate in Counseling and Student Personnel Psychology at the University of Minnesota. During my internship at the Program in Human Sexuality, I became knowledgeable about the theory and techniques of sex therapy. I completed my dissertation of the effects of communication training of the outcome of a sex counseling treatment program. During those early years at the Program in Human Sexuality, I was becoming more aware of a connection between sexuality concerns and chemical dependency. Marilyn Mason, PhD, who trained with me at the Program in Human Sexuality, was responsible for making me more knowledgeable about chemical dependency and sexuality. She was also responsible for helping me look at my personal issues of codependency and was instrumental in encouraging me to go through the family treatment program at Hazelden, Inc., in Center City, Minnesota.

This background led me further to study and to research the connections between sexuality and chemical dependency. In 1979, Philip Colgan, MA and I conducted an informal study of 300 patients seen at the clinic at the Program in Human Sexuality. While we were not surprised to learn that 25% of them had past or current chemical abuse problems, we helped further document that some correlation of sexual problems and chemical dependency existed.

Also in 1979, I formed an advisory board to the Program in Human Sexuality to learn more about the correlation or connection and to consider training opportunities for professionals to become more aware of this connection. The Advisory Board met for a number of years as we implemented teaching programs and I am still indebted to these professionals. They came from a variety of disciplines and were working in chemical dependency agencies, private practice and staff and faculty of the University of Minnesota. It was an exciting group because it drew from so many disciplines and work situations. All had a common bond: each recognized that an important connection between chemical dependency and sexuality was being overlooked by most professionals treating chemical dependency or sexuality problems respectively. Some of these members who attended these meetings were: Jim Bowe (Control Data Corporation), Dagny Christiansen (Granville Programs), Philip Colgan (Program in Human Sexuality), David Dotlick (Honeywell Corporation), Karen Elliot (Hazelden, Inc.), Sue Evans (formerly of Chysalis Treatment Center for Women and then in private practice), Bruce Fischer (Alcohol and Drug Counselor Education Program, University of Minnesota), Miriam Ingribritizen (Family Renewal Center, Fairview-Southdale Hospitals), Judith Justad (CHART), Herb Laube (Program in Human Sexuality), Eleftherious Papageorgiou (St. Mary's Junior College), Jim Schaefer (Office of Alcohol and Other Drug Abuse Programming, University of Minnesota), Sue Schaefer (formerly with Chysalis and Relate and then in private practice), Tom Shroyer (Johnson Institute), Sondra Smalley (formerly with Mercy Medical Center and then in private practice), Terrence Williams (Hazelden, Inc.), and Calvin Vraa (Institute for Psychological Therapies).

One of the first outgrowths of the advisory group was the planning of a National Conference on Chemical Abuse and Sexuality which was sponsored by the Department of Conferences, the Program in Human Sexuality and the Office of Alcohol and Other Drug Abuse Programming (AODAP). In fact, the idea for this conference was given to us by Jim Schaefer, the Director of AODAP. This conference, held in 1980 was an impetus for our next project — to establish a training program to increase the knowledge and skills of chemical dependency practitioners in treating the sexual and intimacy concerns of their clients.

Funding was sought for this program. It fell on deaf ears within the federal funding agencies. However AODAP provided the seeds for the beginning of the training program with the assistance of trainee tuition. In addition, the Program in Human Sexuality, under the direction of the Department Head of Department of Family Practice and Community Health, Edward Ciriacy, MD and the Director of the Program in Human Sexuality, Sharon Satterfield, MD, provided the facilities, the support staff and conceptual support. I would like to thank the administration of the Department and the Program as well as the rest of the faculty and staff for their support of this program over the years. In particular, I would like to thank Diane Campbell and Terry Craig for their administrative support and to John Armour for his media productions and assistance with the media presentations.

AODAP funding subsidized the costs for this program for three years until it became self-supporting through trainee tuition. I am completely indebted to AODAP and particularly to Jim Schaefer and Jim Meland, the Director and Assistant Director, respectively. When we began our summer Institute Program in Chemical Dependency and Family Intimacy, we received scholarship support for many trainees through a generous grant from the Walker Foundation.

AODAP was also instrumental in providing seed funding for a national resource center which provided audiotapes and videotapes of educational material related to Chemical Dependency and Family Intimacy. We received additional funding from the 3M Foundation and DeLuxe Check Printers Foundation.

The training program has continued since that time. The format has changed over the years but the objectives have remained the same. The faculty for the training program were an excellent combination of chemical dependency specialists and sex therapists. The primary faculty were Philip Colgan, MA, Sue Evans, MA, Bruce Fischer, MA, Sandra Nohre, MA, Eleftherious Papageorgiou, MA, Sue Schaefer, MA, Sondra Smalley, MA, and myself. We had numerous guest speakers and some of these were: Robert ten Bensel, PhD, John Brantner, PhD, Miriam Ingebritzen, MSW, Sharon Satterfield, MD, Margretta Dwyer, MA, Peter Bell, John Grace, MSW, and Douglas Elwood, MA. We learned a great deal from each other. And in the process of training hundreds of practitioners over the years, we learned from our trainees.

As a result of our training programs, I feel we have made an important impact on the fields of chemical dependency and sexuality. This volume, in many ways, represents a culmination of what we have learned over the past 6 years of working together. I hope that this volume will further the work we began and continue to help improve the treatment and rehabilitation of chemically dependent individuals and their families.

Eli Coleman, PhD
Associate Professor and Associate Director
Program in Human Sexuality
Department of Family Practice and Community Health
Medical School
University of Minnesota
Minneapolis, Minnesota

Introduction

The causal relationship between chemical dependency and intimacy dysfunction remains poorly understood. Yet the frequency with which these two are linked has become recognized in clinics and treatment centers across the country. The debate about causation of chemical dependency will continue for years. However, if we hope to break the generational cycle of intimacy dysfunction and chemical dependency, the time for effective treatment of these dual disorders is now.

Treatment can only begin when the practitioner clearly understands the total dynamics of intimacy. Intimacy is a qualitative description of a relationship between two or more people. In an intimate relationship, the individuals involved express feelings in a meaningful, constructive, respectful and mutually acceptable manner which leads to the psychological well-being of the individuals involved. Intimate behavior or intimate relationships must include the communication of thoughts and feelings in order to define the boundaries of the relationship and to express feelings of caring, concern and commitment. This communication also helps in the negotiation of roles and rules of the relationship and for resolution of conflicts. Intimate relationships are of varying durations and intensity and are certainly not limited to the parental unit. Intimacy can be found in any type of relationship. Marital intimacy or family intimacy are simply types of intimate relationships. Intimacy can be expressed emotionally, intellectually, socially, sexually, or spiritually and in any combination.

Sexual activity, which is sometimes viewed as synonymous with or as the apex of intimacy, is only an aspect of intimacy and only one method of intimate expression.

Intimacy dysfunction is defined as a developmental or pathological barrier to engaging in intimate behavior. Examples or symptoms of intimacy dysfunction include: physical abuse, emotional neglect, or sexual abuse of children, relationship discord, violent relationships, rape, or psychogenic sexual dysfunction. All of these intimacy dysfunctions have a high correlation with chemical dependency.

Despite the connection between chemical dependency and intimacy dysfunction, the intimacy concerns are rarely recognized in the diagnosis, treatment, and aftercare of the chemically dependent person and his/her family. Often the chemically dependent person has been dependent upon alcohol or other drugs in order to be sexual or to be intimate. Many end up seeking further therapy to deal with sexuality and intimacy issues. Some, however, return to using. Others stay dry but never feel sobriety. Treatment that does not go beyond the control of drinking or other drug abuse and focus on intimacy risks having the chemically dependent person frozen in their insecurity and lacking the skills to develop intimate relationships.

It is the opinion of the editor of this special issue that treatment for intimacy and sexual concerns should be an integral and important consideration in the rehabilitation of the chemically dependent person and their family. Unfortunately, many chemical dependency professionals are unaware of intimacy problems, are unwilling to discuss these issues, or have not received sufficient training to evaluate and treat these issues.

As a result of this lack of training, chemically dependent persons are often discharged from treatment programs still victims of their intimacy dysfunction and chemical dependency. They are also victims of many professionals who have failed to recognize the connection between these two disorders or who have been unable to provide appropriate treatment to this population.

This special charter issue and textbook attempts to give professionals information and skills to deal with intimacy dysfunction issues with the hope of improving treatment and rehabilitation of chemically dependent individuals and their family members. The volume will discuss typical intimacy dysfunctions and treatment methods and strategies which have been found to be effective.

The first three articles by Eli Coleman, PhD, in this volume review the literature which supports the notion that chemical dependency and intimacy dysfunction are inextricably bound. Dr.

Coleman also suggests that this relationship appears to be true for codependency, too. These articles lay the groundwork for the remaining articles in the volume.

As Dr. Coleman points out, shame is an inevitable consequence of intimacy dysfunction. Jeffrey Brown, MSE, provides an excellent review of the literature which links shame, intimacy and sexuality. Besides providing this review of the literature, Mr. Brown makes suggestions for overcoming shame in the therapeutic process. His suggestions are theoretically sound and translated into practical methods which the psychotherapists will find useful.

Another consequence of intimacy dysfunction is boundary inadequacy. Philip Colgan, MA, helps define boundary inadequacy and presents a conceptual approach for skillful assessment of boundary inadequacy. Mr. Colgan suggests that an accurate assessment of patterns of boundary inadequacy and treatment of boundary disorders is an integral part of the successful recovery process of chemically dependent people.

While men and women have both experienced intimacy dysfunction, shame, and boundary inadequacy associated with chemical dependency, less attention has been given in the literature to the sexual and intimacy problems of chemically dependent women. Susan Schaefer, MA, and Sue Evans, MA, discuss the importance of addressing sexuality issues in the treatment of chemically dependent women. Again, this paper provides an excellent review of the existing literature related to this topic as well as providing practical suggestions for incorporating sexuality into the treatment and aftercare of chemically dependent women.

Another neglected issue in the treatment of chemical dependency is the area of sexual orientation concerns. Susan Schaefer, MA, Sue Evans, MA, and Eli Coleman, PhD, discuss the universality of these concerns for chemically dependent men and women despite the general neglect of these issues in treatment. Besides reviewing the supporting evidence for these claims, these authors provide some specific suggestions of what the professional and professional treatment center can do to adequately address this issue in the treatment of chemically dependent men and women.

Sue Evans, MA, and Susan Schaefer, MA, contribute another

important paper to this volume focusing on incest and chemically dependent women. Due to the alarming incidence of incest in the histories of chemically dependent women, this article is particularly important. The experience of incest appears to be a critical variable in the development of intimacy dysfunction for some women and is a critical issue to be addressed in their recovery from chemical dependency. Once again, these authors provide the reader with helpful conceptual and practical suggestions for addressing this issue. In particular, this paper includes an assessment tool which the authors designed for working with incest victims and provides an excellent annotated bibliography as a resource for professionals as well as their clients.

Incest perpetrators and other sex offenders can be found in disproportionate numbers among chemically dependent individuals. Margretta Dwyer, MA, discusses the fact that many sex offenders go undetected by chemically dependent individuals or, if identified, there is the myth that the sex offending behavior will stop once the chemical dependency is treated. Ms. Dwyer provides the professional with a basic understanding of the dynamics of the sex offender and sex offending behavior. She makes suggestions regarding methods of identification, assessment strategies and considerations for choosing an appropriate treatment program for these individuals.

In the next paper, Eli Coleman, PhD, discusses the relationship between chemical dependency, intimacy dysfunction and sexual compulsivity. Sexual compulsivity is a relatively new concept which is beginning to be recognized as a compulsive disorder and is seen in disproportionate numbers among chemically dependent and codependent individuals. Dr. Coleman defines sexual compulsivity and discusses the concerns and the debate about this conceptualization. In addition, he proposes his understanding of the etiological factors and illustrates how similar the development of this disorder is to chemical dependency. Finally, he makes some treatment suggestions which include the importance of identifying these problems, the treatment by appropriately trained professionals, and the importance of providing the client with positive attitudes about sexuality.

Underlying many intimacy dysfunctions are basic problems of codependency. Codependency is found among chemically dependent individuals as well as their family members. Issues of codependency must be addressed to achieve identity and intimacy. Philip Colgan, MA, discusses the treatment of dependency disorders in men. So often, the partners of chemically dependent men are assumed to have problems with dependency. Mr. Colgan suggests that the men he works with often have problems with dependency, identity and intimacy. His paper presents a conceptual framework for understanding dependency disorders in terms of etiology, behavioral manifestations and treatment methodology.

Further discussion of treating codependency and intimacy dysfunctions in dyadic relationships is provided by Sondra Smalley, MA, and Eli Coleman, PhD. Three stages of treatment are identified and illustrated. The results of this therapeutic approach leads to healthy intimacy expression based upon individuation of the clients rather than on compulsive dependent patterns.

More specific treatment suggestions regarding intimacy in recovery are provided by Sandra Nohre, MA. Ms. Nohre focuses more specifically on the sexual functioning aspects of intimacy expression. While the journey toward a healthy sexual lifestyle is dependent upon improvement of self-esteem self-responsibility, communication, touching, and intimacy, sex therapy is shown to be helpful in alleviating sexual dysfunctions as well as enriching the sexual lives of chemically dependent individuals and their partners.

Finally, the last paper included in this volume addresses the general issues of intimacy, aging and chemical dependency. John Brantner, PhD, reviews the essential ingredients of intimacy, discusses the effect of aging on everyone, the impact of chemicals on intimacy and aging, and finally offers some suggestions to the recovering individual regarding these issues. Dr. Brantner's paper summarizes, in many ways, the intent of this volume and ends the volume with some general treatment guidelines.

Thus completes the volume and provides the professional with a comprehensive look at chemical dependency and intimacy dysfunction.

Eli Coleman, PhD

Chemical Dependency and Intimacy Dysfunction: Inextricably Bound

Eli Coleman, PhD

SUMMARY. Despite the fact that chemical dependency and intimacy dysfunction are inextricably bound, intimacy concerns are rarely addressed in the diagnosis, treatment or aftercare of the chemically dependent person or his or her family members. This article is intended to provide information which will help professionals recognize the connection between intimacy concerns and the drug abuse and dependency problems of their clients—and consequently, help them improve the treatment and rehabilitation of those clients.

Despite the fact that chemical dependency and intimacy dysfunction are inextricably bound, intimacy concerns are rarely addressed in the diagnosis, treatment or aftercare of the chemically dependent person and his or her family members. Chemical dependency counselors too often fail to recognize the role that intimacy dysfunction plays in chemical abuse and dependency. The result? Some individuals never attain sobriety because a comprehensive approach to their problem has been overlooked. Other individuals who attain sobriety or responsible use, are often frozen in insecurity and continue to fail in their attempt to develop intimate relationships. They are left with intimacy dysfunctions

---

Dr. Coleman is the Associate Director and Associate Professor at the Program in Human Sexuality, Department of Family Practice and Community Health, Medical School, University of Minnesota, 2630 University Ave. S.E., Minneapolis, MN 55414.
 Reprint requests may be obtained by contacting the author at the address listed above.
 The author would like to acknowledge the assistance of Orlo Otteson in preparing the manuscript.

© 1987 by The Haworth Press, Inc. All rights reserved.

that interfere with successful rehabilitation and the development of feelings of well-being.

And chemically dependent individuals who are being treated for sexual and intimacy concerns are often thwarted in their treatment by therapists who also fail to recognize the link between chemical abuse or dependency and intimacy dysfunction.

It has only been in the past ten years or so, that allied health professionals have had a growing realization of the important connection between chemical abuse and problems related to sexuality and intimacy (see Coleman, 1982 and O'Farrell, Weyland, and Logan, 1983 for reviews of the literature supporting this connection). This article and other articles in this volume is (are) intended to provide chemical dependency counselors and therapists who treat sexual and intimacy problems the information which will help them recognize the connection between intimacy concerns and the drug abuse and dependency problems of their clients—and, consequently, help them improve the treatment and rehabilitation of those clients.

DEFINITIONS

Before the relationships between chemical abuse, dependency and related sexual and intimacy dysfunctions are explored, some working definitions will be offered.

Chemical Abuse

An abusive pattern is defined as the unhealthy use of mood-altering chemicals (e.g., alcohol, marijuana). Examples of unhealthy patterns are: (1) the consistent use of chemicals to maintain "normal" functioning, (2) the dependence on chemicals to produce positive feelings about self, (3) the dependence on chemicals to feel relaxed, (4) an inability to "control" one's use of drugs, (5) and a loss of control of socially accepted behavior while under the influence of drugs (e.g., violence, drunk driving). Chemical abuse can also be defined as the use of psychoactive drugs, in any amount or frequency that interferes with normal functioning and/or significantly causes departure from social norms.

Chemical Dependency

Chemical dependency could be defined as a pattern of use in which the individual experiences harmful consequences and/or preoccupation and/or loss of control over the amount or frequency of use. Chemical dependency is a term that encompasses alcoholism and/or drug dependency. The individual may be psychologically and/or physically dependent on a drug. (Note that in these definitions of abuse, dependency or addiction, the amount of use is not specified.) A common myth is that in order to be considered chemically dependent a chemically dependent person must drink or use all day, everyday. The consequences of use are the criteria used in determining abuse or dependency.

Codependency

Codependency can be defined as an easily identifiable (overt) or carefully disguised (covert) learned pattern of exaggerated dependency and extreme and painful external validation, with resulting identity confusion. The pattern can contain several traits (characteristics) or a single state (a fundamental relationship interaction). See Smalley and Coleman (1987) and Colgan (1987) for a more complete description of codependency.

Intimacy

Intimacy is a qualitative description of a relationship between two or more people. In an intimate relationship, the individuals involved have the ability to express feelings (both positive and negative) in a meaningful and constructive manner and in a way that is mutually acceptable and respectful and that leads to the psychological well-being of the individuals involved. In order to engage in intimate behavior or to be involved in an intimate relationship, one must be able to communicate thoughts and feelings. The purpose of this communication is to define the boundaries of the relationship and to express feelings of caring, concern, and commitment. The purpose is also to negotiate roles and rules of the relationship and to resolve conflicts. Intimate relationships can be of different durations and intensity and are certainly not limited to the parental unit. Intimacy can be found in any kind of relationship: marital intimacy or family intimacy are simply two forms of an intimate relationship. Intimacy can be expressed emotionally, intellectually, socially, sexually, recreationally, vocationally, and spiritually.

Sexual Activity

Sexual activity, which is sometimes viewed as the apex of intimacy, is only a way of expressing intimacy. Sexual activity can be devoid of intimacy (e.g., rape) or be an expression of intimacy. Intimacy can also be expressed without sexual activity (e.g., non-sexual friendship).

Sexuality

Sexuality is a broader concept than intimacy or sexual activity. Our sexuality encompasses our physical, gender, sex-role, and sexual orientation identity—and our physical attractions and our needs for warmth, tenderness, touch, and love. We are sexual in all we do, and therefore our sexuality is always a part of our intimacy or sexual activity.

Intimacy Dysfunction

Intimacy dysfunction is a developmental or pathological barrier to engaging in intimate behavior or relationships. It can take the form of (1) physical abuse, emotional neglect, or sexual abuse of children, (2) psychosexual disorders such as sex offending behavior, (3) relationship or marital discord as a result of conflict, violence, codependency, sexual identity disorders, confusion or conflict in roles, communication problems, unhealthy attitudes regarding sexual activity and intimacy, and sexual dysfunction. All of these intimacy dysfunctions have been found to be highly correlated with chemical abuse and dependency.

THE CORRELATIONS AND RELATIONSHIPS OF INTIMACY DYSFUNCTION AND CHEMICAL ABUSE AND DEPENDENCY

Child Abuse and Neglect

Numerous studies have documented the correlation between various forms of child physical abuse and/or neglect and chemical abuse and/or dependency. These studies indicate a strong relationship between families in which children are abused or neglected and the presence of an alcoholic parent.

Also in examining the literature on the abusing parent, a striking pattern emerges: abusing parents were themselves abused, or neglected, physically or emotionally as children (Spinetta and Rigler, 1972).

Chemical dependency professionals, while initially hesitant, are becoming increasingly aware of the amount of physical abuse and neglect which occurs among chemically dependent families and in children of chemically dependent parents.

They have also become aware of another serious form of child abuse: the abuse of alcohol by the pregnant mother resulting in fetal alcohol syndrome (FAS) (Coles, Smith, Fernhoff, and Falek, 1985; Clarren and Smith, 1978; Strissguth, Herman, and Smith, 1978).

Sexual abuse is another form of child abuse. While the exact incidence of sexual abuse in the histories of chemically dependent persons is not known, various studies have indicated that between 40-70% of chemically dependent women have experienced incest in their childhood. There seems to be a high positive correlation between incest experiences in childhood and later onset of psychiatric, chemical abuse or dependency and psychosexual dysfunctions (see Coleman, 1987a and Evans and Schaefer, 1987 for a review of this literature).

Perpetrators of incest are also commonly found to be alcoholic (e.g., Virkunnen, 1974; Dwyer, 1987). The perpetrators of incest have often experienced an early sexual trauma that has contributed to his or her aberrant behavior (Dwyer, 1987).

The relationship between incest, chemical dependency and

family intimacy dysfunction is not totally clear. These relationships are more closely examined in the article by Coleman 1987a which is included in this volume. Correlations have been found, but the impact of various types of incest on different individuals is difficult to predict. While the relationships are not totally clear, if one of these factors is found to be present, this factor represents a high enough risk for the professional to carefully look to see if the other factors exist and to explore the relationship among them. This may be critical to the understanding of the client's problem as well as the improved chances for successful rehabilitation.

Marital-Relationship Problems

Chemically dependent persons commonly experience difficulties in close relationships. Marital and relationship problems abound. Underlying many of these intimacy difficulties are problems with codependency (see Coleman, 1986; Smalley and Coleman, 1987b; and Colgan 1987 for a more careful review of the problems of codependency).

Other barriers to successful relationships include (1) the inability to clarify or maintain appropriate roles in the relationship, (2) sexual identity conflicts, (3) poor communication skills, (4) unhealthy intimacy and sexual attitudes and values, (5) sexual dysfunction, and (6) violence. (These barriers are fully explored by Coleman, 1987.)

Family Conflict

Disturbed family functioning in the family of origin of chemically dependent individuals has been commonly identified by researchers and clinicians (e.g., Cork, 1969; Hecht, 1973). These types of disturbances are also observed in the current family functioning of chemically dependent individuals (Jacob, Favorini, Meisel, and Anderson, 1978; Orford, Oppenheimer, Egert and Hensman, 1977; Burton and Kaplan, 1968; Bailey, Haberman and Alksne, 1962; Lemert, 1960; Jackson, 1954; Kaufman, 1986; Root, 1986; Whitley and Zankowski, 1986).

Disturbances in family conflict may precede the development of chemical dependency. For example, using a cybernetic paradigm for understanding addictive drinking, Schwartzman (1985) asserts that alcoholism can be perceived as the "solution" to the paradoxical psychosocial context within which they find themselves, to which their addictive drinking is an adaptive response. Many of these alcoholics find the psychosocial context of Alcoholics Anonymous to provide a better "solution" and an aid to changing the psychosocial context of the family functioning.

Other Addictive Disorders

The correlation between chemical dependency and other addictive disorders (e.g., addictive or addictive-like gambling, sexual activity, spending, binge or purge eating, dieting, exercising, etc.) has not been carefully documented. However, there is a growing awareness that there are some significant correlations and that there are more similarities than differences between various addictive disorders (Oxford, 1985). It is the author's hypothesis that family intimacy dysfunction is also highly correlated with these other addictive disorders. This hypothesis has not yet been tested, except currently with a study underway by the author on sexually compulsive individuals. The results of this study are still being analyzed. The important point here is that the possibility exists that family intimacy dysfunction might play a significant part in the etiology or in the consequence of these addictive disorders. Treatment, then, must take this into consideration if rehabilitation is to be effective and complete.

Sexual compulsivity, can become a coping mechanism or an anesthetic (like chemicals) to the psychological pain caused by family intimacy dysfunction. Like a quick "fix," sex becomes a way of shoring up damaged self-esteem or creating a false sense of intimacy. On the other hand, compulsive sexuality can develop patterns of intimacy dysfunction.

Chemically dependent individuals can develop patterns of sexual compulsivity before treatment—or replace chemicals with sexual compulsivity after treatment. Individuals who become sexually compulsive use compulsive sexual activity as a replacement for intimate relationships. Examples of sexual compulsivity include compulsive fetishes, masturbation, or indiscriminate sexual activity. A man, for example, who spends hours a day in adult book stores and who leaves job responsibilities and intimate relationships behind is a good example of someone who has developed a pattern of sexual compulsivity. Just as chemicals formed an intimacy barrier and caused further intimacy dysfunction, sexual compulsivity can do the same. (For more description of this disorder, see Carnes, 1983, 1986; Coleman, 1986; Coleman, 1987.)

Treatment of sexual compulsivity or other addictive or addictive-like disorders is often as difficult as the treatment of chemical dependency. Fortunately, we are understanding these disorders better by understanding the similarities to chemical dependency and other compulsive disorders — and their accompanying intimacy dysfunctions. It is also important for chemical dependency professionals to recognize other addictive or compulsive disorders in their clients. If these other disorders are not treated, the individual is likely to continue to experience disruption in his or her personal/social life and continue to experience intimacy dysfunction.

WHAT DO THESE CORRELATIONS MEAN?

Correlations and relationships have been found to exist between chemical dependency and child abuse, marital-relationship discord, family conflict, and other addictive disorders. What is the cause? Does chemical dependency lead to intimacy dysfunction? Or does intimacy dysfunction lead to chemical dependency? So far, the aforementioned reports reveal correlations and do not imply a cause-effect relationship. This "chicken or egg" type of question, however, is answered by the integrated model, Figure 1, that was first illustrated by Coleman (1983) and then further elaborated by Coleman and Colgan (1986). The cycle can begin at any point; the starting point is irrelevant because of the long standing pattern that is passed on from generation to generation. Disturbed family dynamics and individual intimacy dysfunctions are an inevitable consequence of chemical dependency. This leads to intimacy dysfunction in the family and boundary inadequacy in individuals. In order to better cope and retain family stability, there is an increased need for alcohol and chemical abuse. With unhealthy expressions of intimacy in the family,

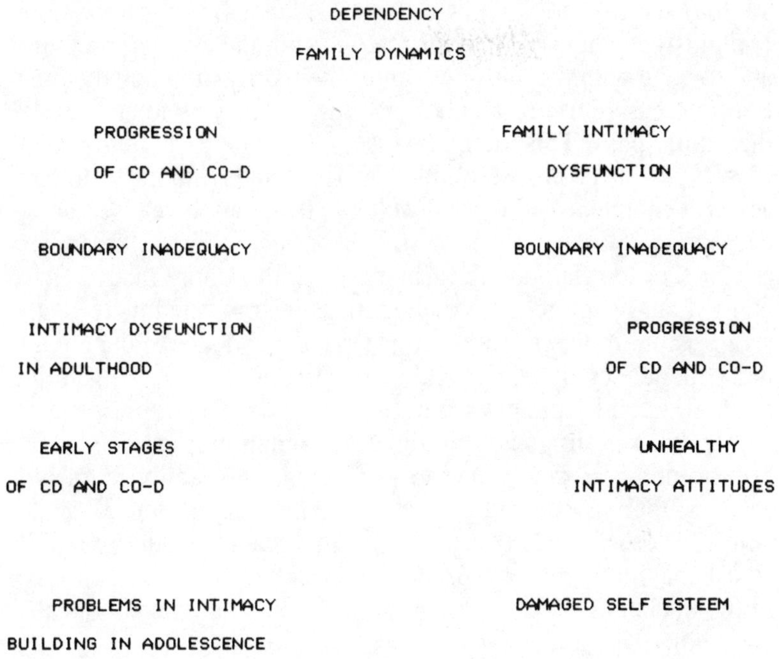

```
                        DEPENDENCY
                      FAMILY DYNAMICS


        PROGRESSION                    FAMILY INTIMACY
        OF CD AND CO-D                   DYSFUNCTION


     BOUNDARY INADEQUACY              BOUNDARY INADEQUACY


     INTIMACY DYSFUNCTION                PROGRESSION
        IN ADULTHOOD                   OF CD AND CO-D


        EARLY STAGES                     UNHEALTHY
        OF CD AND CO-D                INTIMACY ATTITUDES


     PROBLEMS IN INTIMACY             DAMAGED SELF ESTEEM
   BUILDING IN ADOLESCENCE


                   LACK OF INTIMACY MODELS
```

Figure 1. Interactive Model of Chemical Dependency
           and Family Intimacy Dysfunction

sexual attitudes are developed in the children that are based on the parental role models. As the chemical dependency patterns progress, there is damage to the self-esteem of family members. With a lack of healthy sexual and intimacy attitudes, a lack of healthy role models, boundary inadequacy and a lowered self-esteem, the child tries to develop intimate and sexual relationships in adolescence and adulthood. With these handicaps and developmental deficiencies, it is little wonder that the adolescent has difficulty. This process inhibits the normal psychosocial and psychosexual development. In an Eriksonian (Erikson, 1968) sense, unsuccessful resolution of early developmental stages occurs that prevents further resolution of developmental stages in adulthood. The adolescent turns to alcohol or drugs (or other compulsive behavior patterns) to cope with the existing pressures and to cope with the chronic pain of the family intimacy dysfunction. Excessive use of alcohol or drugs is one way to anesthetize the family pain. This method is used to feel better about oneself. However, this positive feeling is artificial and temporary. In fact, as the dependency pattern develops, it begins to cause further damage to intimacy patterns and self-esteem. Thus, the adolescent enters adulthood with further problems with intimacy. There is, then, a greater need for coping mechanisms, and this feeds the progression of dependency. This dependency leads to the continued dependency dynamics and begins the process again, handing down this family pattern from generation to generation.

Alcohol and drugs are not the only coping mechanisms which family members can utilize to anesthetize the family pain. Nor are they the only behaviors that cause intimacy problems to develop. Excessive use of sex, food, or work, — or other compulsive behaviors — may be used. Codependent behaviors are also found in chemically dependent families, and these behaviors also are compulsive and serve the same function.

CONCLUSION

Families are affected by chemical dependency in a profound way. As indicated in the intimacy model, this is a vicious cycle that is passed from generation to generation. Intimacy skills and attitudes are developed by children in families that are dysfunctional. Boundary confusion and invasion create boundary inadequacy in adulthood. If we are going to break the vicious cycle of intimacy dysfunction, we need to address intimacy issues of all family members. Claudia Black (1981) has described enormous negative effects on self-esteem and intimacy functioning in the children of alcoholic parents. These children need help. We must go beyond the rehabilitation of the chemically dependent person and his or her partner and deal also with family members. ("Family" may not always mean children, as in the case of lesbian and gay male relationships.) We must expand our definition of family to include close, significant relationships.

We need to examine some of the same intimacy issues of the chemically dependent individual and look at other family members. What sexual and intimacy attitudes have they formed? Do they feel shameful about themselves? Do they know what their boundaries are, how to set them, and how to respect others? How comfortable are they with their own sex role identity? Have they developed rigid sex role behavior? What are their concerns about sexual preference? What sexual functioning concerns do they have? What compulsive sexual habits have they developed? How do they communicate with their friends, with family members, and in sexual relationships? Do they have a healthy balance of independence-dependence in relationships? These questions need to be asked and the problems addressed. This will reduce the likelihood that these family members will need to find addictive behaviors to shore up self-esteem, to anesthetize pain, to be sexual, and to feel intimate.

Despite the fact that chemical dependency and intimacy dysfunction are inextricably bound, intimacy concerns are rarely addressed in the diagnosis, treatment, or aftercare of the chemically dependent person and his/her family. Treatment must go beyond the control of drinking or other drug abuse and deal with the intimacy issues. Upon obtaining sobriety, or responsible use, a person is often frozen in insecurity and lacking the skills to develop intimate relationships. Often the chemically dependent person is dependent upon alcohol or other drugs in order to be sexual or to be intimate. For many, the chemical use is controlled, but they often need more. Many seek out further therapy to deal with sexuality and intimacy issues. Some return to using. Others stay dry but never feel sober.

The behavioral and reeducation approaches of sex therapy have been very helpful to many individuals in recovery. This type of therapy lends itself well to those with developmental deficits, since the terms of intimacy expression are based upon egalitarian values, assertive philosophy, open expression of feelings, pleasure focused sex and boundary setting.

In addition, therapists are treating individuals with sexual concerns need to recognize the potential for alcohol and other drug abuse. Many sex therapists have not only avoided looking at the chemical use pattern of their clients but also have encouraged chemical use as part of therapy. There are very few educational sex therapy films that do not involve some chemical use. The couples in these films are often sipping wine, smoking cigarettes or using some chemical before or after sex. Physicians have treated many sexual problems with a prescription of a tranquilizer or by telling the patient, "Just have a drink before you go to bed and relax." Treatment for sexual concerns should not begin until the problem of chemical abuse has been addressed—and treated, if necessary.

Treatment for intimacy and sexual concerns should be an integral and important consideration in the rehabilitation of the chemically dependent and codependent individual. Unfortunately, many professionals in the field of chemical dependency are unaware of the kinds of intimacy problems that exist, are unwilling to discuss or deal with these issues, and/or have not received sufficient training required to effectively know how to refer or treat these issues. This is the reason the Program in Human Sexuality pioneered training efforts to teach professionals working in the field of chemical dependency to deal more effectively with intimacy issues of their clients.

In the meantime, many individuals are left with intimacy dysfunctions that serve as a barrier to successful rehabilitation and to greater feelings of well-being and sobriety. These individuals are not only the victims of intimacy dysfunction and chemical dependency, but they are also victims of professionals who have failed to see the connection between these two dynamics and who have been unable to provide appropriate services to this population. Fortunately, there are more and more professionals who are concerned and aware and who are asking questions and dealing with these issues. This special issue which is devoted to chemical dependency and intimacy dysfunction, attempts to give the professional more information and skills to deal with intimacy issues and dysfunction and, consequently, to improve treatment and rehabilitation of chemically dependent and codependent individuals and their family members.

REFERENCES

Bailey, M. B., Haberman, P. & Alksne, H. 1962. Outcomes of alcoholic marriages: Endurance, termination or recovery. *Quarterly Journal of Studies on Alcohol*, Vol. 23: 610-623.
Black, C. 1981. *It Will Never Happen to Me*. Denver: M.A.C. Publications.
Burton, G. & Kaplan, H. M. 1968. Sexual behavior and adjustment of married alcoholics. *Quarterly Journal of Studies on Alcohol*, Vol. 29: 603-609.

Carnes, P. 1983. *Out of the Shadows: Understanding Sexual Addiction*. Minneapolis, Minnesota: Compcare Publications.

Carnes, P. 1986. Progress in sexual addiction: An addiction perspective. *SIECUS Report*. Vol. *14*(6): 4-6.

Claren, S. K. & Smith, D. W. 1978. The fetal alcohol syndrome. *New England Journal of Medicine*. Vol. *298*: 1063-1067.

Coleman, E. 1982. Family intimacy and chemical abuse: The connection. *Journal of Psychoactive Drugs*, Vol. *14*: 153-158.

Coleman, E. 1983. Sexuality and the alcoholic family: Effects of chemical dependence and co-dependence upon individual family members. In P. Golding (Ed.) *Alcoholism: Analysis of a World-wide Problem*. Lancaster, England: MTP Press.

Coleman, E. 1986. Sexual compulsion vs. sexual addiction: The debate continues. *SIECUS Report*. Vol. *14*(6): 7-11.

Coleman, E. 1987a. Child physical and sexual abuse among chemically dependent individuals. *Journal of Chemical Dependency Treatment*. Vol. *1*.

Coleman, E. 1987b. Marital and relationship problems among chemically dependent and codependent individuals. *Journal of Chemical Dependency Treatment*. Vol. *1*.

Coleman, E. & Colgan, P. 1986. Boundary inadequacy in drug dependent families. *Journal of Psychoactive Drugs*. Vol. *18*: 21-30.

Coleman, E. 1987c. Sexual compulsivity: Definition, etiology, and treatment considerations. *Journal of Chemical Dependency Treatment*. Vol. *1*.

Coles, C. D., Smith, I., Fernhoff, P. M., & Falek, A. 1985. Neonatal neurobehavioral characteristics as correlates of maternal alcohol use during gestation. *Alcoholism: Clinical and Experimental Research*. Vol. *9*: 454-460.

Colgan, P. 1986. Treatment of dependency disorders in men: A balance of identity and intimacy. *Journal of Chemical Dependency Treatment*. Vol. *1*.

Cork, M. R. 1969. *The Forgotten Children*. Toronto: Paperjacks, in association with the Addiction Research Foundation.

Dwyer, M. 1986. Identifying the male chemically dependent sex offender and a description of treatment models. *Journal of Chemical Dependency Treatment*. Vol. *1*.

Erikson, E. H. 1968. *Identity: Youth and Crisis*. New York: Norton.

Evans, S. & Schaefer, S. 1986. Incest and chemically dependent women: Treatment implications. *Journal of Chemical Dependency Treatment*. Vol. *1*.

Hecht, M. 1973. Children of alcoholics. *American Journal of Nursing*. Vol. *73*: 1764-1767.

Jackson, J. 1954. The adjustment of the family to the crisis of alcoholism. *Quarterly Journal of Studies on Alcohol*, Vol. *15*: 562-586.

Jacob, T., Favorini, A., Meisel, S. S. & Anderson, C. M. 1978. The alcoholic's spouse, children and family interactions: Substantive findings and methodological issues. *Journal of Studies on Alcohol*, Vol. *39*: 1231-1251.

Kaufman, E. 1986. A workable system of family therapy for drug dependence. *Journal of Psychoactive Drugs*. Vol. *18*: 43-50.

Lemert, E. M. 1960. The occurrence and sequence of events in the adjustment of families to alcoholism. *Quarterly Journal of Studies on Alcohol*. Vol. *21*: 679-697.

O'Farrell, T. J., Weyland, C. A., & Logan, D. 1983. *Alcohol and Sexuality: An Annotated Bibliography on Alcohol Use, Alcoholism, and Human Sexual Behavior*. Phoenix, Arizona: Oryx Press.

Orford, J. 1985. *Excessive Appetites: A Psychologist's View of Addictions*. New York: John Wiley & Sons.

Orford, J., Oppenheimer, E., Egert, S. & Hensman, C. 1977. The role of excessive drinking in alcoholism complicated marriages: A study of stability and change over a one-year period. *International Journal of Addictions*. Vol. *12*: 471-495.

Root, L. E. 1986. Treatment of the alcoholic family. *Journal of Psychoactive Drugs*. Vol. *18*: 51-56.

Schwartzman, J. 1985. Alcoholics anonymous and the family: A systemic perspective. *American Journal of Drug and Alcohol Abuse*. Vol. *11*: 69-89.

Smalley and Coleman, E. 1987. Treating intimacy dysfunctions in dyadic relationships among chemically dependent and codependent relationships. *Journal of Chemical Dependency Treatment*. Vol. *1*.

Spinetta, J. J. & Rigler, D. 1972. The child abusing parent: A psychological review. *Psychological Bulletin*. Vol. *77*: 2966-304.

Streissguth, A. P., Herman, C. & Smith, D. 1978. Intelligence, behavior, and dysmorphogenesis in FAS: A report on two patients. *Journal of Pediatrics*. Vol. *92*: 363-366.

Virkkunen, M. Incest offenses and alcoholism. 1974. *Medical Science and the Law*. Vol. *14*: 124-128.

Whitely, M. J. & Zankowski, G. L. Family therapy in a hospital setting: A model for time-limited treatment. *Journal of Psychoactive Drugs*. Vol. *18*: 61-64.

Child Physical and Sexual Abuse Among Chemically Dependent Individuals

Eli Coleman, PhD

SUMMARY. Numerous studies have documented the correlation between various forms of child physical abuse and/or neglect, sexual abuse, other sex offending behavior and chemical abuse and/or dependency. In treating any of these disorders, professionals should be aware of the high risk of interrelatedness of these factors and that in addition to addressing relevant factors, the underlying dynamics of intimacy dysfunction, shame, and boundary inadequacy need to be treated.

CHILD PHYSICAL ABUSE AND NEGLECT

Intimacy dysfunction is a developmental or pathological barrier to engaging in intimate behaviors or relationships (Coleman, 1987). One of the examples or symptoms of intimacy dysfunction is child abuse and neglect. Numerous studies have documented the correlation between various forms of child physical abuse and/or neglect and chemical abuse and/or dependency. Although the exact correlations do not exist, the interactive relationship between child physical abuse and neglect, chemical

---

Dr. Coleman is the Associate Professor at the Program in Human Sexuality, Department of Family Practice and Community Health, Medical School, University of Minnesota, 2630 University Ave. S.E., Minneapolis, MN 55414.

Reprint requests may be obtained by contacting the author at the address listed above.

The author would like to acknowledge the assistance of Orlo Otteson in preparing the manuscript.

© 1987 by The Haworth Press, Inc. All rights reserved.

abuse or dependency, and family intimacy dysfunction are abundantly clear. The incidence varies up to 84% (Cohen and Densen-Gerber, 1982) depending upon the study. One of the larger studies (Young, 1964) examined 300 families in which children had been abused and neglected and found that drinking was a "primary family problem" in 62% of the families and that "heavy drinking" was present although not the primary problem, in other additional families. In a more recent study (Cohen and Densen-Gerber, 1982), social histories were collected on 178 patients who were being treated for drug/alcohol addiction. Eighty-four percent reported a history of child abuse and neglect including experiences of incest and rape.

These studies indicate a strong relationship between child abuse or neglect and the presence of an alcoholic parent. Some of the evidence suggests that neglect is more prevalent than physical abuse. In spite of these alarming correlations, some professionals continue to ignore the relationship between chemical dependency and child physical abuse and neglect (e.g., Strauss, 1979).

The literature on the abusing parent shows a striking pattern: abusing parents were themselves abused or neglected, physically or emotionally, as children (Spinetta and Rigler, 1972). In their review of the literature, Spinetta and Rigler concluded that ". . . the child is the father of the man. The capacity to love is not inherent; it must be taught to the child. Character development depends on love, tolerance, and example. Many abusing parents were raised without this love and tolerance." And yet, in their review of the literature, the researchers did not consider the relationship between chemical dependency and child abuse and neglect.

But many chemical dependency professionals are becoming increasingly aware of the degree of physical abuse and neglect that occurs in chemically dependent families and among children of chemically dependent parents. Robert ten Bensel, MD, MPH, a national expert in the area of child abuse and neglect, has stated the case emphatically: "By definition, where there is alcoholism existing in a family, the emotional neglect of children is occurring."

FETAL ALCOHOL SYNDROME

Another form of physical child abuse that has more recently been documented is the abuse of alcohol by the pregnant mother that results in fetal alcohol syndrome (FAS). Symptoms of FAS include dysmorphic features, growth retardation, and central nervous system damage that causes mental retardation and other persistent alterations in development and behavior (Coles, Smith, Fernhoff, and Falek, 1985; Clarren and Smith, 1978; Streissguth, Herman, and Smith, 1978). In one study, intrauterine growth failure occurred with increasing use of alcohol during pregnancy. While alcohol use and abuse has been more closely related to FAS, the behavior of infants is similar to that reported for infants exposed to other central nervous system depressants like heroin and methadone (Finnegan and MacNew, 1974; Finnegan, 1975; Finnegan and Fehr, 1980). These effects can be better treated and prevented when the issues of chemical use are addressed in prenatal medical care (Connaughton, Reeser, Schut, and Finnegan, 1977). For a more detailed summary of the effects of drug dependence in pregnancy, see Finnegan (1979).

Child physical abuse (neo- and perinatally) affects children in serious ways. The abuse is clearly related to serious negative effects on the child (much of which is not fully understood because of the lack of longitudinal studies). The negative physical effects are clearly visible in the neonatal child but not all effects are visible and other negative effects might be lifelong. Although this kind of abuse causes clear physical harm to the child, child abuse laws do not protect the developing fetus.

SEXUAL ABUSE

Sexual abuse is another form of child abuse. In 1975, Benward and Densen-Gerber reported that among 118 female patients treated for chemical dependency, 44% had been victims of incest. Treatment centers throughout Minnesota that have informally polled chemically dependent women have found 40-50% of these women have had childhood incest experiences (Evans and Schaefer, 1980). Sterne, Schaefer, and Evans (1983) reported that 46% of a sample of 75 chemically dependent women experienced incest in their family histories. A study conducted by Weiss in 1977 found that 70% of adolescent females treated for chemical dependency experienced incest. An accurate estimate of incest experiences among chemically dependent women is difficult to make. These studies cited showed a range between 40-70%. These are startling findings and they emphasize the need to further examine the problem and to address it in the treatment and aftercare of these women (Evans and Schaefer, 1987).

These findings should be viewed in the context of the general demographic statistics that are available. Studies on non-clinical populations regularly show that between 15-30% of women and 5-10% of men have been sexually victimized as children (Finkelhor, 1979; Gagnon, 1965). The incidence for chemically dependent women is at least 100% greater than in the general population.

Women who have experienced incest seem also to be at risk for the development of other psychiatric problems. For example, Emslie and Rosenfeld (1983) reported that in a study of 65 children and adolescents who were hospitalized for psychiatric problems, 37.5% of the nonpsychotic girls had a history of incest; 10% of the psychotic girls had such a history, as did 8% of the 39 psychotic and non-psychotic boys. This study and others (e.g., Browning and Boatman, 1977; Herman and Hirschman, 1981) consistently describe severe family disorganization, with resulting ego impairment in the incest families; and this family disorganization may account for more of the damage to the ego development of the child than the incest experience. As Browning and Boatman show, the typical family constellation is that of a chronically depressed mother, an alcoholic and violent father or stepfather, and an eldest daughter who is forced to assume many of her mother's responsibilities, with ensuing role confusion.

Besides psychiatric and psychosexual dysfunctions that seem to result from incest experiences (e.g., Linberg and Distad, 1985), many women treated for incest have alcohol or drug-related problems. For example, at the Program in Human Sexuality, we have found that approximately 30% of women treated for family sexual abuse have been chemical abusers or were chemically dependent (Colgan and Coleman, 1979).

The relationship between chemical dependency and incest in

males is not known. In the past, there has been a tendency to view only females as victims, and rarely were questions asked of males. Many of us are starting to ask these questions, and we have been surprised and shocked to find as many cases as we do. This question has not been systematically investigated and needs to be. There is a likelihood that a relationship will be found.

The relationship between incest, chemical dependency, and family intimacy dysfunction is not totally clear. Correlations have been found but the impact of various types of incest on different individuals is difficult to predict. Finkelhor and Browne (1985) have provided a framework for a more systematic understanding of the effects of child sexual abuse. They identified four traumagenic dynamics as the cause of core psychological injuries. These dynamics are (1) traumatic sexualization, (2) betrayal, (3) stigmatization, and (4) powerlessness. In their view, stigmatization contributes most to the development of chemical abuse or dependency problems. In this dynamic, stigmatization grows out of the child's prior knowledge that incest is taboo, and it is certainly reinforced when, if disclosed, people react with shock or hysteria or blame the child for what has transpired. Traumatic sexualization is most likely to lead to sexual disorders and dysfunctions. The other dynamics lead to different psychological results and behavioral manifestations, none of which seem to contribute to positive mental health. These problems can indirectly lead to chemical abuse problems or barriers to intimacy functioning.

SHAME

One of the inevitable consequences of physical abuse, neglect, or sexual abuse is the development of feelings of shame. Shame is a feeling of unworthiness or sinfulness—or a feeling of being unwanted (see Kaufman, 1980; Brown, 1987; Evans and Schaefer, 1987 for a more thorough discussion of this dynamic). Shame inhibits an individual from feeling worthy of an intimate relationship. Feelings of shame are a result of some type of family intimacy dysfunction. Unloved, neglected, or abused individuals feel bad or sinful about most every aspect of their personhood. Many chemical dependency and sex therapy professionals have become well aware of this dynamic, and they realize the presence of shame as the main symptom in those who have experienced family intimacy dysfunction and the main cause of continued intimacy dysfunction and compulsive behaviors in adulthood. Resolution of these feelings are essential in the recovery process.

BOUNDARY INADEQUACY

One of the other inevitable consequences of family intimacy dysfunction is boundary inadequacy. Boundary inadequacy has been defined as a pattern of ambiguous, overly rigid, or invasive boundaries that are related to physical or psychological space (Coleman and Colgan, 1986). Boundary inadequacy can be both a precursor and a result of chemical dependence (Coleman, 1983). Coleman and Colgan (1986) found that in a sample of 122 alcoholic and 187 non-alcoholic subjects the alcoholic sample reported more boundary inadequacy while growing up. These childhood experiences created pain and difficulties in interpersonal relationships and in the formation or maintenance of intimate relationships. Lack of personal boundaries, overly rigid boundaries, or lack of respect for others' boundaries are seeds for intimacy dysfunction. Skills at boundary setting play an essential role in developing and maintaining healthy intimate relationships (Coleman and Colgan, 1986). See Colgan (1987) for a more thorough description of boundary inadequacy and treatment strategies to alleviate these difficulties.

Developing skills at boundary setting is an essential ingredient in the recovery from chemical dependency or codependency. For many it is learning to say "no" to someone's request for physical, sexual or emotional intimacy. Through saying "no," the individual learns that he or she can have a personal boundary and have it respected. This leads to a clear sense of self-wants and self-desires and it develops a sense of power and control in interpersonal relationships. After learning to say "no," the individual can learn to say "yes" and not lose a sense of individuality.

Learning to respect boundaries is another necessary step or

function. While some chemically dependent individuals have not learned to set or defend personal boundaries, others have learned to disrespect or invade boundaries. For this second group of individuals, "no" only means "try harder." Learning to ask for intimacy and to respect "no" is a skill that all recovering individuals need.

PERPETRATORS OF INCEST

Perpetrators of incest are a good example of individuals who have problems dealing with intimacy dysfunction and boundary inadequacy — in particular lacking the skills at boundary setting and respecting anothers' personal boundaries. In 1974, Virkkunen reported that of 45 cases of incest studied, 49% of the male perpetrators were found to be alcoholic. At the sex offender treatment program at the University of Minnesota, 90-95% of incest fathers have been found to be alcoholic or were periodically abusing alcohol at the time of their offenses (Dwyer, 1987). Dwyer notes that the incidence of chemical abuse or dependency among pedophiles is significantly lower than among incest perpetrators. This indicates that the chemically dependent person is at high risk for incest perpetration and the children are at risk for victimization. Even among female alcoholics, there is an increased risk for incest perpetration. Sterne, Evans and Schaefer (1983) reported that 8% of their sample of 75 chemically dependent women indicated they had sexually abused at least one of their own children.

The perpetrator of incest has often experienced an early sexual trauma that has contributed to his or her aberrant behavior. Approximately 56% of 130 sex offenders treated at the Program in Human Sexuality reported having been sexually abused as children (Dwyer, 1987). Finkelor and Browne (1985) have also indicated that a number of traumagenic dynamics of child sexual abuse can lead victims to abuse their own children or to allow their own children to be victimized by others.

Once again, a significant correlation between incest perpetration, chemical abuse or dependency and family intimacy dysfunction can be seen. Although the relationships are not totally clear, when one of these dynamics is present, there is a high probability that the other factors also exist.

In addition to incest perpetrators, it should be noted that various other sex offenders (e.g., exhibitionists, voyeurs, child molesters, obscene phone callers, rapists) have significant correlated problems with chemical abuse and dependency. Approximately 30% of the sex offenders treated at the Program in Human Sexuality in 1979 had been found to be chemically dependent (Colgan and Coleman, 1979). In a more recent study of 140 sex offenders treated at the Program in Human Sexuality, 33% were diagnosed with chemical dependency (Dwyer, Amberson, and Seabloom, 1985), a percentage that is consistent with the previously conducted study.

Dwyer et al. also reported that 56% of these sex offenders reported that they were sexually abused as children (although the authors thought the men underestimated this incidence). Family disorganization and lack of intimacy was found to be almost universal, and current psychological and interpersonal and inter-familial functioning was also found to be significantly impaired.

Pedophiles

In other studies, a high percentage of alcoholism and problem drinking has been found in child molesters. Rada (1976) reported that of 203 male child molesters, 49% were drinking at the time of commission of the offense, and 34% of this group were drinking heavily. On the basis of the Michigan Alcoholism Screening Test (MAST), 52% were rated as alcoholic.

These findings suggest that alcohol may play an important role in the commission of these offenses. Rada suggests that the use of alcohol lowers inhibitions and facilitates commission of an offense that is much less likely to occur in the sober state. He also suggests that as alcoholism removes these individuals further and further from acceptable adult sexual objects the child becomes an attractive sexual outlet. Impotence and decreased testosterone levels, he says, are also a secondary effect of alcohol abuse and would lead to forms of regressed sexual contact with children. Rada concludes that the child molester needs ongoing treatment not only for his sexual difficulties but for his alcohol abuse. However, treatment programs have traditionally tended to focus on only one aspect of the problem (one or the other), and it is rare to find programs that address both problems.

Rapists

As a crime of violence, it is no surprise to find high rates of alcohol and drug abuse and dependency among rapists. Rada (1975) reported that of 77 incarcerated male rapists 50% had been drinking at the time of the rape, and 35% were found to be alcoholic by MAST standards. In another study, Groth (1979) found that of 500 rapists 40% had a history of alcohol abuse, and alcohol was involved in the majority of these rape incidents. Rada (1975) believes that unlike the child molester the rapist does not drink to lower inhibitions; rather he drinks to increase his sense of confidence and power prior to commission of the offense. Groth's study also found that a third of the sample had been sexually traumatized when they were children. Most of these men had been victimized as children by female family members, a common experience among rapists—the victim becomes the victimizer.

James Prescott (1975), a neuropsychologist, believes that the principal cause of human violence is a lack of bodily pleasure during the formative periods of life. Laboratory experiments and cross-cultural surveys, he says, demonstrate that individuals and societies that experience and promote physical pleasure also tend to be peaceful. In the author's clinical experience, many sex offenders, especially the violent ones, were denied physical bodily pleasures as children and were more likely to be neglected or abused.

The incidence of chemically dependent individuals having raped someone or having been raped has not been documented—nor has the incidence of marital rape been investigated. It is the author's clinical experience, however, that the incidence of marital rape is especially high among chemically dependent couples and that this is a serious issue in the recovery process.

CONCLUSION REGARDING SEX OFFENDERS

Removing alcohol from sex offenders who have abused alcohol does not eliminate the sex offending behavior, a mistake that many chemical dependency treatment centers make. It is assumed that once the alcohol or drug abuse is under control, the individual will not commit these "deviant" acts. This is not true. The individual might do it less, might do it more, or might do it at the same rate. Rarely, if ever, does the behavior disappear altogether. Many individuals who seek treatment and have been involved in sex offending behavior wish for such an instantaneous cure. When they realize they haven't lost the desire for the sex offending behavior, they become discouraged and despairing. Many look for psychic relief by returning to alcohol and other drugs. At least when using, they had a "good excuse" for their behavior.

CONCLUSION

The interactive relationship between child physical abuse and neglect, family sexual abuse, sex offending behavior, intimacy dysfunction and alcohol and drug abuse and dependency are abundantly clear. In treating any of these disorders, the professional must be aware of the high risk that one or more of the other disorders also exist. Successful or total rehabilitation is contingent on being aware of the inextricably bound nature of these disorders and consequently a more complete treatment approach.

REFERENCES

Benward, J. & Densen-Gerber, J. 1975. Incest as a causative factor in anti-social behavior: An exploratory study. *Contemporary Drug Problems* Vol *4*: 323-340.

Brown, J. 1987. Shame, intimacy, and sexuality. *Journal of Chemical Dependency Treatment* Vol *1*.

Browning, D. H. & Boatman, B. 1977. Incest: children at risk. *American Journal of Psychiatry* Vol *134*: 68-72.

Claren, S. K. & Smith, D. W. 1978. The fetal alcohol syndrome. *New England Journal of Medicine* Vol *298*: 1063-1067.

Cohen, F. S. & Densen-Gerber, J. 1982. *Child Abuse and Neglect* Vol 6: 383-387.

Coleman, E. 1983. Sexuality and the alcoholic family: Effects of chemical dependence

and co-dependence upon individual family members. In P. Golding (Ed.) *Alcoholism: Analysis of a World-Wide Problem*. Lancaster, England: MTP Press.
Coleman, E. 1987. Chemical dependency and intimacy dysfunction: Inextricably bound. *Journal of Chemical Dependency Treatment* Vol *1*.
Coleman, E. & Colgan, P. 1986. Boundary inadequacy in drug dependent families. *Journal of Psychoactive Drugs* Vol *18*: 21-30.
Coles, C. D., Smith, I., Fernhoff, P. M. & Falek, A. 1985. Neonatal neurobehavioral characteristics as correlates of maternal alcohol use during gestation. *Alcoholism: Clinical and Experimental Research* Vol 9: 454-460.
Colgan, P. 1987. Assessment and treatment of boundary inadequacy in chemically dependent individuals and families. *Journal of Chemical Dependency Treatment* Vol *1*.
Colgan, P. and Coleman, E. 1979. *Chemical dependency among patients treated for sexual concerns*. Informal study conducted at the Program in Human Sexuality, University of Minnesota Medical School, Minneapolis, Minnesota.
Connaughton, J. F., Reeser, D., Schut, J., & Finnegan, L. P. 1977. Perinatal addiction: Outcome and management. *American Journal of Obstetrics and Gynecology* Vol *129*: 679-686.
Dwyer, M. 1987. Identifying the male chemically dependent sex offender and a description of treatment models. *Journal of Chemical Dependency Treatment* Vol *1*.
Dwyer, M., Amberson, I. J., & Seabloom, W. 1985. *A theoretical base for a sex offender treatment program*. Unpublished manuscript.
Emslie, G. J. & Rosenfeld, A. 1983. Incest reported by children and adolescents hospitalized for severe psychiatric problems. *American Journal of Psychiatry* Vol *140*: 708-711.
Evans, S. & Schaefer, S. 1980. Why women's sexuality is important to address in chemically dependent treatment programs. *Grassroots: Treatment and Rehabilitation* September: 37-40.
Evans, S. & Schaefer, S. 1987. Incest and chemically dependent women: Treatment implications. *Journal of Chemical Dependency Treatment* Vol *1*.
Finkelhor, D. 1979. *Sexually Victimized Children*. New York: Free Press.
Finkelhor, D. & Browne, A. 1985. The traumatic impact of child sexual abuse: A conceptualization. *American Journal of Orthopsychiatry* Vol *55*: 530-541.
Finnegan, L. P. 1975. Narcotics dependence in pregnancy. *Journal of Psychedelic Drugs* Vol 7: 299-311.
Finnegan, L. P. (Ed.). 1979. *Drug Dependency in Pregnancy: Clinical Management of Mother and Child*. Washington, D.C.: DHEW Publication No (ADM) 79-678.
Finnegan, L. P. & Fehr, K. 1980. The effects of opiates, sedative-hypnotics, amphetamines, cannabis, and other psychoactive drugs on the fetus and newborn. In O. J. Kalant (Ed.) *Alcohol and Drug Problems in Women*. New York: Plenum Press.
Finnegan, L. P. & MacNew, B. 1974. Care of the addictive infant. *American Journal of Nursing* Vol 74: 685-693.
Gagnon, J. 1965. Female child victims of sex offenses. *Social Problems* Vol *13*: 176-192.
Groth, N. 1979. *Men Who Rape*. New York: Plenum.
Herman, J. & Hirshman, L. 1981. Families at risk for father-daughter incest. *American Journal of Psychiatry* Vol *138*: 967-970.
Kaufman, G. 1980. *Shame: The Power of Caring*. Cambridge: Shenkman.
Kinsey, B. A. 1966. *The Female Alcoholic: A Sociological Study*. Springfield, Ill.: Thomas.

Kogan, K. L. & Jackson, J. K. 1963. Role perceptions in wives of alcoholics and of nonalcoholics. *Quarterly Journal of Studies on Alcohol.* Vol. *24*: 627-639.

Lindberg, F. H. & Distad, L. J. 1985. Survival responses to incest: Adolescents in crisis. *Child Abuse and Neglect* Vol *9*: 521-526.

Prescott, J. W. 1975. Body pleasure and the origins of violence. *The Futurist* Vol April: 64-74.

Rada, R. T. 1976. Alcoholism and the child molester. *Annals of the New York Academy of Sciences.* Vol *273*: 492-496.

Rada, R. T. 1975. Alcoholism and forcible rape. *American Journal of Psychiatry* Vol *132*: 444-446.

Spinetta, J. J. & Rigler, D. 1972. The child abusing parent: A psychological review. *Psychological Bulletin* Vol. *77*: 2966-304.

Strauss, M. 1979. Family patterns and child abuse in a nationally representative sample. *Child Abuse and Neglect* Vol *3*: 213-225.

Streissguth, A. P., Herman, C., & Smith, D. 1978. Intelligence, behavior, and dysmorphogenesis in FAS: A report on two patients. *Journal of Pediatrics* Vol *92*: 363-366.

Sterne, M., Schaefer, S. & Evans, S. 1983. Women's sexuality and alcoholism. In P. Golding (Ed.) *Alcoholism: Analysis of a World-Wide Problem.* Lancaster, England, MTP Press Limited.

ten Bensel, R. 1981. *Child abuse and neglect: An overview.* Lecture given to Chemical Dependency and Family Intimacy Training Program, Program in Human Sexuality, University of Minnesota Medical School.

Virkkunen, M. 1974. Incest offenses and alcoholism. *Medical Science and the Law* Vol *14*: 124-128.

Young, L. 1984. *Wednesday's Children: A Study of Child Neglect and Abuse.* New York: McGraw-Hill.

Marital and Relationship Problems Among Chemically Dependent and Codependent Relationships

Eli Coleman, PhD

SUMMARY. There is a growing awareness that the marital and relationship problems must be addressed and worked upon if the chemically dependent person is going to maintain his or her sobriety. The involvement of the spouse or partner is important because of the family system dynamics that caused, perpetuated, and/or enabled the chemical dependency needs to be addressed and all involved need some treatment. Recognizing the source of marital or relationship discord is helpful in determining the chemically dependent and codependent couple's needs in terms of aftercare or therapy needed to resolve these conflicts. This article reviews the common problems encountered by many chemically dependent and codependent couples: codependency, sexual identity conflicts, violence in their relationship, confusion in roles, communication difficulties, unhealthy sexual and intimacy attitudes and values and sexual dysfunctions. Essentially, the chemically dependent or codependent couple is experiencing intimacy dysfunction and is often lacking in intimacy skills. These skills need to be learned in order for them to experience intimacy and to feel more complete in their sobriety.

Fear of intimacy and intimacy dysfunction is closely related with chemical dependency and codependency. It is little wonder that marital relationship problems exist so frequently among

---

Dr. Coleman is the Associate Director and Associate Professor at the Program in Human Sexuality, Department of Family Practice and Community Health, Medical School, University of Minnesota, 2630 University Ave. S.E., Minneapolis, MN 55414.
Reprint requests may be obtained by contacting the author at the address listed above.
The author would like to acknowledge the assistance of Orlo Otteson in preparing the manuscript.

© 1987 by The Haworth Press, Inc. All rights reserved.

chemically dependent and codependent individuals; issues of trust, communication, loyalty, commitment, and jealousy abound. This fact has been documented by a number of studies (Coleman, 1982b; Paolino and McCrady, 1977; Rae and Drewery, 1972; Gorad, 1971; Paredes, 1973; Burton and Kaplan, 1968; Bailey, Haberman, and Alksne, 1962; Bailey, 1961; Smalley & Coleman, 1986). It is also known that incidence rates of divorce are much higher than what is found in the "normal" population (Lisansky, 1957; Kinsey, 1966). More husbands of alcoholic women leave their wives than do wives of alcoholic men leave their husbands (Mandel and North, 1982).

CODEPENDENCY

Smalley and Coleman (1987) and Colgan (1987) argue that therapists must address the underlying codependency traits in order to begin resolving the intimacy dysfunctions experienced by chemically dependent individuals and their partners in order to begin resolving the intimacy dysfunctions. Chemically dependent couples need each other in unhealthy ways: they either begin their relationship because of their codependency or develop it because of the needs created by the chemical dependency. Having been unloved, neglected, or abused creates a need for human warmth, caring, and touch that is often beyond fulfillment. As one client put it,

> I can never seem to convince John that I love him. He needs to be constantly touched and reassured. I have to tell him I love him twenty times a day. He doesn't want to go anywhere without me. I am his only true friend. I feel completely responsible for his well-being.

Another way of dealing with codependency is to create distance. As another client put it, "If I don't get close to anyone, I can't get hurt. I won't lose myself and get confused." Distance is a coping mechanism for codependency. Some couples swing back and forth between intense closeness and complete distance.

Their codependency on each other acts as a magnet that can attract as well as repel with great force.

Keeping a rigid distance or maintaining a suffocating closeness are methods for coping with codependency. Depending on the type of codependency problem and how it manifests itself, solutions are available. Assignments that bring about more separateness or togetherness can be given in treatment to bring about more balance in the system. For example, a very enmeshed couple should attend different AA or Alanon groups in different buildings and at different times. Disengaged couples need to experience activities together.

Most chemical dependency professionals seem simply to understand the marital or relationship difficulties as a result of living in a chemically dependent situation. However, previous experiences and personality disturbances can contribute to chemical abuse problems (e.g., incest experiences that lead to poor ego functioning and cause a person to develop a relationship with a chemically dependent person). Wives of alcoholics have been described as either submissive and as having poor ego strength (e.g., Kogan and Jackson, 1963; Mitchell, 1959; and Lemert, 1962) or dominant (e.g., Whalen, 1953). However, Hurwitz and Daya (1977) note that wives of alcoholics who do not seek help present themselves as dominant persons—a façade for basic codependency. Therefore, most wives probably possess some elements of codependency that are sometimes carefully disguised as dominance, independence, and/or strong ego functioning. Smalley and Coleman (1987) and Colgan (1987) caution the practitioner not to underestimate the codependency traits that exist in the chemically dependent person or his or her partner. Both individuals may appear to be compulsively dependent or independent, in either case demonstrating faulty ego functioning that ultimately provides a significant barrier to intimacy expression. This overt contradiction might explain why some partners of chemically dependent individuals (especially the compulsively independent type) might appear psychologically normal based upon empirical testing in comparison to controls (e.g., Paolino, McCrady, Diamond, and Longabaugh, 1976) while other clinical reports describe a contrary picture (e.g., Edwards, Harvey, and

Whitehead, 1973; Price, 1945; and Lewis, 1945). No psychometric instrument seems able to identify the characteristics of codependency as described by many chemical dependency professionals (Smalley and Coleman, 1987). And, yet, many practitioners are well aware of the dual problems that exist in these relationships and understand that not all the problems can be attributed to the effects of living in a chemically dependent situation—although some can. This is why many practitioners begin to see the difficulties of the partner of the chemically dependent person only after the chemically dependent partner stops using chemicals and begins to develop better ego functioning. Or, it also explains why many chemically dependent persons do not develop better ego functioning simply as a result of abstaining from the use of chemicals. In some cases, abstinence exacerbates the problem.

SEXUAL IDENTITY CONFLICTS

In order to be intimate with another human being, it is important to have an established identity—which codependency precludes. Also a lack of clear and positive identity development may result in codependency, chemical dependency, and family intimacy dysfunction. Codependency, chemical dependency, and family intimacy dysfunction interrupts positive sexual identity development. So, in order to be intimate with another human being, it is also important to have a sexual identity about which one feels positive.

One's sexual identity is composed of one's physical, gender, sex role, and sexual orientation identity.

Physical and Gender Identity

Gender identity involves one's knowledge of oneself as male or female. Confusion of this gender identity is referred to as gender dysphoria and may lead to transsexualism and the desire of the individual to change his or her physical identity in order to match it with his or her own gender identity. These cases are few in number, but it has been the experience at the Program in Human Sexuality that a high percentage of these people have concomitant chemical abuse or dependency problems.

Sex Role Identity

Sex role identity involves one's identity with traditional sex role stereotypes. Chemically dependent and codependent individuals are often unable to feel good about their masculinity or femininity. Researchers have indicated that many people drink or use chemicals to deal with the disparity between one's ideal sex role image and one's actual sex role image. Sandmaier (1980) has confirmed what other researchers (Wilsnack, 1976; and Schucket, 1972) have found regarding the relationship of sex roles and chemical use/abuse. Sandmaier found in interviewing 50 recovering alcoholic women that these women fell into one of two patterns, depending on their conscious acceptance or rejection of traditional feminine stereotypical roles. Both acceptance and rejection of these gender-determined roles created stress for them and contributed to their chemical dependency. The disparity between what they were, what they wanted to be, and what they thought they should be caused stress, and this stress was relieved by drinking.

McClelland, Davis, Kalin, and Wanner (1972) found that men often drink to feel more masculine. Drinking gives them a sense of personal power, control, or mastery. Other males, however, who feel restricted by male sex role stereotypes use alcohol or drugs to engage in behaviors that are stereotypically feminine (e.g., expressing feelings, crying, embracing a friend, etc.).

For men and women, the struggle for comfort with a sex role identity produces the stress that alcohol or drugs temporarily relieve. The double bind is that abuse leads to worsened feelings about one's masculinity or femininity. "A man should be able to hold his liquor." "It's not lady-like to be drunk."

Research has not documented the link between sex roles and codependent behavior patterns. However, the author sees from a clinical perspective that many codependent individuals are struggling with these same sex role issues (see Colgan, 1987; and Smalley and Coleman, 1987).

Many chemically dependent and codependent individuals hold on to rigid sex role behaviors or maintain a rigid rejection of sex role behavior as a way of coping with insecurities of sex role identities. They are afraid to express a mixture of masculine and feminine behavior for fear they will be less of a man or a woman.

The pressures created by sex role standards, or the confusion created by changing sex role standards, are a definite part of the etiology and/or the damage created by chemical dependency and codependency. Although the use of chemicals may make an individual feel better about sex role identity, when the individual loses control of alcohol or drug use or develops more serious codependent behavior patterns, his masculinity or her femininity is questioned. An alcoholic or drug addict feels less of a man or a woman and feels that he or she can no longer fulfill the roles they or society would like them to fulfill.

Mandel and North (1982) argue that sex role issues must be dealt with in the treatment of chemically dependent women. They also suggest that treatment for women cannot be based upon the treatment mode designed for men. They cite the underutilization of services and poorer success rates for women as an indication that different treatment programs need to be developed (see Schaefer and Evans, 1987).

Treatment methods designed for men have addressed, to some degree, sex role issues. The emphasis that is placed on the expression of feelings, expression of affection to other men, and the value men's groups have all, at least indirectly, addressed a number of male sex role issues. Even so, more direct attention to sex role issues is needed for men (see Colgan, 1987).

In dealing with chemically dependent and codependent men and women, it is helpful to teach the concept of androgyny. A sexually healthy person is one who can express the traditionally masculine and feminine role behaviors and still feel good about himself or herself as a male or a female. For example, we teach men they can cry, express emotion, and be nurtured and supported; but they can also be strong, dominant, and care-taking. Women can be strong, assertive, and in charge as well as soft, caring, and emotional. It is individuals who feel trapped by their sex roles who feel less masculine or feminine.

Sex Orientation Identity

As one component of sexual identity, chemically dependent and codependent individuals are almost all concerned about sexual preference. Concerns, insecurity, doubt, and fears about sexual preference can inhibit intimacy with people, regardless of gender. These concerns and feelings can be a source of anxiety, guilt, shame, and discomfort. For some, fear of being or becoming homosexual is an ongoing concern or an unconscious fear. Closeness to same-sex individuals can lead to confusion about these feelings. Thoughts of past homosexual activity can cause confusion, discomfort, guilt, and shame. Even an awareness of a same-sex fantasy or dream is enough to generate stress.

There are also those with predominate same sex attractions who have evaded these feelings through the use of alcohol or drug abuse. They have denied these feelings and have used these behavior patterns to help them forget. Others have acted on these feelings, felt shame about them, and used alcohol or drugs to mask the shame. Many individuals who are going through treatment for chemical dependency and who have identified themselves as homosexual prior to treatment, invariably feel the guilt and shame about their homosexuality once alcohol or drugs are removed.

There have been varying estimates about the degree of chemical abuse problems among the gay and lesbian populations (e.g., Fifield, Latham, & Philips, 1978). These researchers reported that 30% of the homosexual community have some problems with alcohol. Disturbed family relationships are often seen as the cause of homosexuality. This is an erroneous assumption, as the research by Bell, Weinberg, and Hammersmith (1981) has found. Often, the disturbed familial relationships are a result of the awareness of homosexuality in the child. Also, homosexuals with disturbed familial backgrounds are more likely to come to the attention of the professional community. It is also this group that is most likely to develop chemical abuse and dependency problems.

Oppression, alienation, guilt, shame, and disturbed family relationships all contribute to self-abusive patterns and lead naturally to alcohol and drug abuse problems. The gay and lesbian community also uses bars as a setting for socializing. For many, there are few alternatives to socializing in bars, and this factor also contributes to the abusive pattern.

Alcohol and drugs so easily serve as a coping mechanism for dealing with the stigma of homosexuality and the difficulties of achieving intimacy in a predominately heterosexual society. When sober and homosexual, the individual is faced with the task of embracing his or her homosexuality and developing self-acceptance and the skills to function in intimate relationships in a predominately heterosexual society that oppresses homosexuality.

At the Program in Human Sexuality, we encourage individuals to deal directly with their homosexual feelings and behavior as part of their recovery process. Homophobia is an "illness" that prevents intimacy in any intimate relationship whether it be same sex or opposite sex. It is helpful for individuals in recovery to be exposed to openly gay and lesbian individuals, to be educated about the myths of homosexuality-bisexuality, and to talk among themselves about homosexual feelings and behavior (see Evans, Schaefer, & Coleman, 1987 for more discussion of this issue).

VIOLENCE IN RELATIONSHIPS

Violence is an obvious symptom of intimacy dysfunction and obviously a cause, as well, of intimacy dysfunction. It is often correlated with chemical abuse or dependency. Violence in relationships in the general population is not as uncommon as we might like to believe. Beginning in courtship, a number of studies indicate that between 16-30% of couples experience some form of violence in their relationship (Makepeace, 1981, 1983; Cate, Henton, Kaval, Christopher, and Lloyd, 1982; Bernard and Bernard, 1983). In an attempt to improve on the methodology of these studies through better random sampling, Murphy (1984) found an even higher incidence of violence—40.4%. Murphy also found that the family environment (whether or not violence occurred) predisposes an individual toward physical and sexual abuse in his or her dating relationship.

Over six million incidents of serious physical abuse occur in families each year (Strauss, 1979). Violence is not an isolated phenomenon that affects only one victim in the family (Hindman, 1979). The "battering family" is an apt phrase since it is likely that more than one victim and perpetrator exists in the family. For example, abused wives may also be child abusers (Scott, 1974).

What contributes to this phenomenon? Langley and Levy (1977) cite alcohol and drugs—particularly alcohol—as the major contributor (see Hamilton and Collins, 1981 for a review of this literature). Roy (1977) reports that the husband's alcohol and other drug abuse was the underlying factor in over 80% of the cases reported to the Abused Women's Aid in Crisis (AWAIC) in New York City. Of the men involved in relationships exceeding seven years duration, 90% were reported to have had alcoholic and other drug problems. Husbands in this group did not have to be drunk or on drugs when committing a violent act; many times the assaults occurred during sobriety or when the effects of the drugs had worn off (Roy, 1977). These alarming findings have been also supported by Carder (1978). In a survey of 100 wives of alcoholics, none of whom were identified as victims of marital violence, 72% of the women reported that they had been physically threatened, 45% had been beaten, and 27% described potentially lethal assaults (Scott, 1974). Gelles (1974), however, is quick to point out that not all the violence is caused by drinking. Again, this intimacy disorder is to some degree independent of chemical abuse or dependency. Although highly correlated, one cannot assume that when drinking stops the violence will diminish. This certainly occurs; however the opposite can also occur.

The other factor that seems to contribute to family violence is a history of violence between parents—usually in the form of the father assaulting the mother—and the physical and/or sexual abuse of the women in these families as children. The husbands are also likely to have experienced emotional deprivation, lack of protection, and violence both as witnesses and as abused children (Hilberman and Munson, 1977/78).

Again, in a study of 100 cases of wife battering, Gayford (1975) found a high incidence of family violence in the families of both partners, and drunkenness and previous imprisonment among the husbands. There was also an association found between wife battering and child abuse.

Violence is all too common in chemically dependent and codependent relationships. It is one of the obvious symptoms of intimacy dysfunction and a cause of intimacy dysfunction. In helping couples restore intimacy in their relationship, the issue of past or current violence must be addressed. Deep feelings of hurt and hostility will prevent a couple from working toward a closer, intimate relationship with each other.

CONFUSION OF ROLES IN THE RELATIONSHIP

Another negative consequence of chemical dependency and intimacy dysfunction is the confusion of roles which often develops in the relationship. Parades (1973) has described alcoholic marriages as a

> . . . hotly contested battle of the sexes in which each spouse is not quite sure of which role they represent. The wife seems to ask herself, "Shall I be a mother, companion, or marriage partner to this man?" The husband seems to be unable to decide whether to play the role of the wife's child, her companion, or her husband.(p. 106)

He also describes the interaction pattern that is seen in relationships of the alcoholic man and his wife. The wife has to look after his primary needs as a mother would do with her child. A mother-child relationship develops. The husband becomes more incapacitated as the illness progresses and fits more and more into a childlike helpless role.

Role reversals, role confusion, role inconsistency—all these contribute to a distorted relationship. Sobriety is often stressful because the relationship usually has accommodated and adapted to the pathological state. The disturbed relationship still tries to maintain the system. A dramatic change such as sobriety threatens the stability of the relationship. The individuals are faced with the task of changing their roles in order to accommodate and adjust to sobriety. Some partners do not want to give up their adopted roles. For example, a wife who has learned to be the breadwinner and decision-maker for the household may not want to give up that role. During the drinking days, the alcoholic depends upon the wife to maintain that role. During sobriety, the alcoholic would like to retrieve at least part of the role he abandoned. Many divorces occur after one to two years of sobriety, a result of many problems of intimacy, but a result also of the couples' failure to find or redefine roles of the relationship that can successfully accommodate sobriety or non-codependent behavior.

Couples need to examine roles that were employed while using/abusing chemicals and then define new roles for themselves in sobriety. This adjustment can occur through the general support of AA, Alanon, or couples growth groups at treatment centers. For others, the battle of roles persists, and more intensive therapy is needed.

COMMUNICATION DIFFICULTIES

One of the first casualties of the development of chemical dependency is good communication in relationships. For some, good communication never existed. Because of negative communication patterns witnessed while growing up, an individual may have never learned healthy and positive communication skills. For others, the progression of chemical dependency quickly destroys any meaningful and constructive communication. The progression of the illness causes greater defensiveness, self-centeredness, dishonesty, blaming, and withdrawal. Individuals stop communicating with themselves and thus have little to say to others. Negative experiences with communication reinforce the need not to communicate. Violation of boundaries leads to resentment and the desire to punish the other (e.g., physical or sexual abuse, or other forms of violence). Non-communication is seen as a punishing tool. All these mechanisms and many more serve to destroy good communication.

Treatment centers have been addressing marital and relationship problems more directly by involving the spouse or partner of the chemically dependent person. Aftercare in many treatment centers today relies upon a couples growth group in addition to AA and Alanon groups. The emphasis of groups in AA, Alanon,

Alateen and treatment centers does much to improve the communication skills of its members and clients; some need additional help. Once codependency, identity and sexual identity issues and issues of violence are addressed, together with the problem of confusion of roles in relationships, many clients benefit from learning communication skills — such as attending a four-week class on improving interpersonal communication skills (Couples Communication Program — CCP). The methods in this program attempt to increase communication, openness, and honesty. Through communication, trust and understanding are developed.

INTIMACY AND SEXUAL ATTITUDES AND VALUES

When basic problems related to codependency, sexual identity concerns, violence, confusion in roles, and communication have been addressed, couples are ready to examine their intimacy and sexual attitudes and values. Also before a couple is ready to work on their sexual lives and their intimacy, it is helpful for them to examine their existing attitudes and values, understand where they came from, and to learn attitudes and values that promote healthy sexual functioning and intimacy rather than those that serve as a barrier to it. Intimacy dysfunction stems from, in part, unhealthy attitudes about sexuality, sexual activity, and intimacy. The author has found in his clinical practice that chemically dependent couples often have unhealthy sexual and intimacy attitudes that they so often have learned from their families of origin. Attitudes about sexual activity and intimacy that the author has found frequently in his clinical practice among chemically dependent families are:

"Intimacy doesn't exist."
"Intimacy is something you only have when chemicals are involved."
"Intimacy is something you take; it is never given freely."
"You can only be intimate if there is sex involved."
"Sex can never be associated with intimacy."
"Sex is dirty."
"Seductive behavior gets you want you want."

"Sex will give you power."
"Sex will make you feel powerless."
"Men only want sex."
"Women are frigid."

One predominant attitude that is often found and that was described earlier is feelings of shame. Not only do many feel a basic sense of unworthiness, sinfulness, or being unloved, but they also possess a feeling of shame about their sexual feelings. Alcohol or other drugs are often used to overcome shame in order to be sexual. Many adolescents begin using alcohol or other drugs at the same time they are learning to be sexual with others. Adolescents with shame-based personalities, or with shameful feelings about their sexuality, need alcohol or other drugs to be sexual. Others need drugs or alcohol as an excuse or mechanism to avoid sex in order to avoid their shameful feelings. Either way, intimacy expression or avoidance of intimacy is always associated with chemical abuse or dependency. Chemicals help mask or avoid shameful feelings.

When the use of chemicals stop, the coping mechanism for shame is removed. The individual becomes inundated with feelings of shame about sexuality or sexual activity. So in recovery, shameful feelings usually surface, and the individual needs to overcome his or her shame or find some other coping mechanism. Some stop having sex, and others develop sexual dysfunctions. Others function sexually but cut off their feelings from the activity. So many clients at the Program in Human Sexuality feel like "sexual cripples" following chemical dependency treatment. They are afraid, insecure, and uncertain. Ironically, then, chemical dependency treatment often causes an individual to experience sexual difficulties. Or, at least, they feel disappointed that chemical dependency treatment has not improved their sex lives. These attitudes serve as barriers to healthy intimacy and sexual expression.

The most important attitudes that many sex therapists teach in their clinical practices are:

"Intimacy is based upon openness, honesty, communication, and respect for one another."

"There are many different ways of expressing intimacy other than through sexual activity, all of which are important."
"Sex does not have to be associated with guilt."
"Every person should take responsibility for themselves in a sexual relationship."
"Be responsive rather than responsible for our partner's pleasure."
"The biggest sexual organ is our brain and not our genitals."

For some, a positive and healthy perspective of intimacy and sexuality is enough to overcome these shameful feelings (see Brantner, 1987 for more discussion of healthy attitudes regarding intimacy). For others, whose source of shame is a result of physical and/or sexual invasion of their boundaries, as in the case of incest or physical abuse, therapy is needed to "work through" these experiences.

SEXUAL DYSFUNCTION

Finally, chemically dependent and codependent couples are ready to address issues of sexual dysfunction. Once again, the origin of sexual functioning problems in chemically dependent and codependent relationships can be found prior to the onset of chemical dependency, during the course of chemical abuse, or after the cessation of chemical use. Many studies have documented the link between alcoholism or drug abuse and sexual dysfunction (Akhtar, 1976; Smith, Lemere, and Dunn, 1972; Lemere and Smith, 1973; DeLeon and Wexler, 1973; Gay and Sheppard, 1973; Angrist and Gershon, 1972; Greaves, 1972; Wieland and Yunger, 1970; Malatesta, Pollack, Wilbanks, and Adams, 1979). Many drugs—prescription or illicit—will, even at low doses, suppress or inhibit libido, erection, emission, and/or ejaculation in males—and lubrication or orgasm in females. Prescription drugs with known sexual side effects are the antihypertensives (e.g., methyldopa, reserpine, propanolal, thiazide diuretics), antipsychotics (e.g., thioridazine, chlorpromazine, haloperidol), antidepressants (amitriptyline, desipramine, lithium), androgens, antiandrogens, progestins, and estrogens. (See Story, 1974; Renshaw, 1978; Buffum, 1982; and Abel, 1980 for a review of this literature.)

In addition to these commonly prescribed drugs, other drugs that are sometimes prescribed but are more often illicitly used can produce negative sexual side effects. These drugs include the opiates, stimulants, depressants (e.g., alcohol, methaqualone, barbiturates), marijuana, and psychedelics. Alcohol, specifically, has been shown through a number of studies to decrease sexual performance (e.g., Powell, Viamontes, & Brown, 1974) and chronic abuse can temporarily depress or permanently destroy sexual ability (Lemere and Smith, 1973; Akhtar, 1977). It should be noted that many individuals report positive sexual side effects of drug and alcohol use in small doses.

This may be due in part to the interaction with the person's social learning history and the amount of drug ingested. Wilson (1977) has summarized a number of studies (e.g., Wilson and Lawson, 1976a, 1976b; Briddell and Wilson, 1976) which conclude that although there is a consistent dose-related negative physiological effect on genital responses, the importance of social-psychological factors (including the person's expectations) determine the physiological and psychological effect to some degree (see also Rubin and Henson, 1976).

For example, many drugs have been tried as an aphrodisiac; and many individuals will testify to their value. However none of these substances have ever survived the scrutiny of scientific investigation and been found truly to be an enhancer of sexual capacity. Placebo and expectancy effects account for most of the variance between treatment groups.

Pheromones are being investigated currently for possible aphrodisiac characteristics. Androstenol, a pheronome derived from human male sweat, has been used by the perfume industry and found to be very attractive to females. Pheronomes may be the most promising for a true aphrodisiac (Buffum, 1982).

Sexual dysfunction is a common complaint of recovering chemically dependent and codependent individuals and may have a direct bearing on their potential for recovery (Dowsling, 1980; Coleman, 1982a, 1982b; Nohre, 1987). Lack of desire, premature ejaculation, retarded ejaculation, orgasmic dysfunctions, erectile, and lubrication difficulties are common dysfunctions among chemically dependent individuals. These problems may be a direct result of the aforementioned problems of codependency, sexual identity, violence, confusion of roles, communication, and/or attitudes and values. Or these sexual dysfunctions may simply be a result of discomfort and anxiety about sexuality. These dysfunctions can also develop as a result of the disruption of the association of drugs and sexual functioning. When an individual has always relied on drugs in order to be sexual, the removal of this "crutch" leaves the individual a "sexual cripple." The individual needs to learn how to walk again without the "crutch" and deal with the source of shameful, anxious feelings about sexuality. Intimacy dysfunction, negative attitudes about sexuality, shame, past traumatic experiences with sexual activity, lack of sexual education, and anxiety about performance, can all cause or perpetuate sexual functioning difficulties.

Beckman (1979) illustrated in her study of 120 women alcoholics and 119 women non-alcoholics that one reason why some of the women drank was to improve their sense of sexual adequacy. A significant portion of her sample of alcoholic women reported fairly low sexual satisfaction. She concluded that certain beliefs regarding alcohol and sexuality may contribute to the development of alcoholism in women, or excessive drinking may create sexual problems that are then alleviated or denied by additional drinking. These findings have been confirmed by a more recent study of 35 alcoholic women and their paired nonalcoholic counterparts (Covington and Kohen, 1984).

Sexual dysfunctions can also be a result of physiological damage caused by alcohol or other drug abuse (Van Thiel and Lester, 1976). Liver disease and alcoholic hepatitis are particularly responsible for this type of damage. Since the liver is involved in the metabolization of sexual hormones, liver disease will result in altered hormone levels and secondarily will cause sexual difficulties. Pancreas damage due to alcohol abuse will result in diabetes. Diabetes in turn causes erectile dysfunction and vaginal lubrication problems. Circulatory problems may be responsible for this or peripheral neuropathy.

Organic brain damage is another way that alcohol damages the brain and secondarily impairs sexual functioning. Fortunately, we are treating alcoholism and drug addiction in early stages, so this kind of cortical damage is avoided or minimized.

Examination for physical causes of sexual dysfunction is always important in working with chemically dependent individuals. The psychogenic etiologies are often present with organic etiologies, and they very often interact to produce the sexual dysfunction.

Sources of the sexual dysfunction should be carefully examined by a competently trained sex therapist. Depending on the etiology, some sex dysfunctions are easily treated by a sensitive counselor through education and simple suggestions. Other sexual dysfunctions need the care of a competently trained physician or sex therapist (see Nohre, 1987 for more discussion on this issue). Other intimacy dysfunctions discussed earlier in this paper may need to be treated first before problems or sexual dysfunction are resolved.

In conclusion, because of the high correlations that are found between sexual dysfunction and chemical abuse and dependency, sex therapy should be utilized more frequently as part of the recovery process. Sex should be viewed as one of the important ways couples communication and express intimacy (Coleman, 1982b; Dowsling, 1980; and Nohre, 1987).

CONCLUSION REGARDING MARITAL-RELATIONSHIP DIFFICULTIES

It is helpful to understand that chemical dependency is related to intimacy dysfunction in primary relationships. It is also helpful to understand that intimacy dysfunctions do not disappear when chemical use stops. Recognizing the source of marital or relationship discord is helpful in determining the individual couple's needs in terms of aftercare or therapy needed to resolve these conflicts. Essentially, the chemically dependent or codependent couple is often lacking in intimacy skills, and these need to be learned in order for them to experience intimacy and to feel more complete in their sobriety.

Since there is growing recognition that the intimacy needs and problems must be addressed and worked upon if the chemically dependent person is going to maintain his or her sobriety, the involvement of the spouse or partner is important because of the family system dynamics that caused, perpetuated, and/or enabled the chemical dependency needs to be addressed and all involved need some treatment. And, by giving chemically dependent or codependent couples some new rules and some roles to play with each other, there is less need to abuse chemicals or continue codependent patterns in order to maintain this disturbed family system.

REFERENCES

Abel, E. L. 1980. A review of alcohol's effects on sex and reproduction. *Drug and Alcohol Dependence.* Vol. 5: 321-332.
Akhtar, M. J. 1977. Sexual disorders in male alcoholics. In J. S. Madden; R. Walker, & W. H. Kenyon (Eds.) *Alcoholism and Drug Dependence.* New York: Plenum.
Angrist, B. & Gershon, S. 1972. Some recent studies on amphetamine psychosis—unresolved issues. In E. H. Ellingwood and S. Cohen (Eds.) *Current Concepts on Amphetamine Abuse.* Rockville, Maryland: NIMH.
Bailey, M. B. 1961. Alcoholism and marriage: A review of research and professional literature. *Quarterly Journal of Studies on Alcohol.* Vol. 22: 81-97.
Bailey, M. B., Haberman, P. & Alksne, H. 1962. Outcomes of alcoholic marriages: Endurance, termination or recovery. *Quarterly Journal of Studies on Alcohol.* Vol. 23: 610-623.
Beckman, L. J. 1979. Beliefs about the causes of alcohol-related problems among alcoholic and nonalcoholic women. *Journal of Clinical Psychology.* Vol. 35: 663-670.
Bell, A. P., Weinberg, M. S., & Hammersmith, S. K. 1981. *Sexual Preference: Its Development in Men and Women.* Bloomington: Indiana University Press.
Bernard, M. L. & Bernard, J. L. 1983. Violent intimacy: The family as a model for love relationships. *Family Relations.* Vol. 32: 283-286.
Brantner, J. 1987. Intimacy, aging and chemical dependency. *Journal of Chemical Dependency Treatment.* Vol. 1.
Briddell, D. W. & Wilson, G. T. 1976. The effects of alcohol and expectancy set on male sexual arousal. *Journal of Abnormal Psychology.* Vol. 85: 225-234.
Buffum, J. 1982. Pharmacosexology: The effects of drugs on sexual function—A review. *Journal of Psychoactive Drugs.* Vol. 14: 5-44.
Burton, G. & Kaplan, H. M. 1968. Sexual behavior and adjustment of married alcoholics. *Quarterly Journal of Studies on Alcohol.* Vol. 29: 603-609.
Cate, R., Henton, J., Kaval, J., Christopher, S., and Lloyd, S. 1982. Premarital abuse: A social psychological perspective. *Journal of Family Issues.* Vol. 3: 79-91.
Carder, J. H. 1978. *Families in trouble.* Paper presented at 24th International Institute on the Prevention of Treatment of Alcoholism, Zurich.
Coleman, E. 1982a. Family intimacy and chemical abuse: The connection. *Journal of Psychoactive Drugs.* Vol. 14: 153-158.
Coleman, E. 1982b. How chemical dependency harms marital and sexual relationships. *Medical Aspects of Human Sexuality.* Vol. 16: 42n-42ee.
Colgan, P. 1987. Treatment of dependency disorders in men: A balance of identity and intimacy. *Journal of Chemical Dependency Treatment.* Vol. 1.

Covington, S. S. & Kohen, J. 1984. Women, alcohol and sexuality. *Advances in Alcohol and Substance Abuse*. Vol. *4*: 41-56.
DeLeon, G. & Wexler, H. K. 1973. Heroin addiction: Its relation to sexual behavior and sexual experience. *Journal of Abnormal Psychology*. Vol. *81*: 36-38.
Dowsling, J. L. 1980. Sex therapy for recovering alcoholics: An essential part of family therapy. *The International Journal of the Addictions*. Vol. *15*: 1179-1189.
Edwards, P., Harvey, C., & Whitehead, P. C. 1973. Wives of alcoholics; a critical review and analysis. *Quarterly Journal of Studies on Alcohol*. Vol *34*: 112-132.
Evans, S., Schaefer, S. & Coleman, E. 1987. Sexual orientation conflicts among chemically dependent men and women. *Journal of Chemical Dependency Treatment*. Vol. *1*.
Fifield, L., Latham, J. D. & Phillips, C. 1978. *Alcoholism in the gay community: The price of alienation, isolation, and oppression*. Sacramento: California Division of Substance Abuse.
Gay, G. R. & Sheppard, C. W. 1973. Sex-crazed dope fiends! Myth or reality? In E. Harms (Ed.) *Drugs and Youth: The Challenge of Today*. New York: Pergamon.
Gayford, J. J. 1975. Wife battering: a preliminary study of 100 cases. *British Medical Journal*. Vol. *1*: 194-197.
Gelles, R. J. 1974. *The Violent Home: A Study of Physical Aggression Between Husbands and Wives*. Beverley Hills: Sage Publications.
Gorad, S. L. 1971. Communication styles and interaction of alcoholics and their wives. *Family Process*. Vol. *10*: 475-489.
Greaves, G. 1972. Sexual disturbance among chronic amphetamine users. *Journal of Nervous and Mental Disease*. Vol. *155*: 363-365.
Hamilton, C. J. & Collins, J. J. 1981. The role of alcohol in wife beating and child abuse: A review of the literature. In J. J. Collins (Ed.) *Drinking and Crime*. New York: Guilford Press.
Hilberman, E. & Munson, K. 1977/78. Sixty battered women. *Victimology*. Vol. *2*: 460-470.
Hindman, M. 1977. Child abuse and neglect: The alcohol connection. *Alcohol Health and Research World*. Vol. *1*: Spring.
Hurwitz, J. I. & Daya, D. K. 1977. Non-help-seeking wives of employed alcoholics: A multilevel interpersonal profile. *Journal of Studies on Alcohol*. Vol. *38*: 1730-1739.
Kinsey, B. A. 1966. *The female alcoholic: a sociological study*. Springfield, IL: Thomas.
Kogan, K. L. & Jackson, J. K. 1963. Role perceptions in wives of alcoholics and of nonalcoholics. *Quarterly Journal of Studies on Alcohol*. Vol. *24*: 627-639.
Langley, R. & Levy, R. C. 1977. *Wife Beating*. New York: Dutton.
Lemere, F. & Smith, J. W. 1973. Alcohol-induced sexual impotency. *American Journal of Psychiatry*. Vol. *130*: 212-213.
Lemert, E. M. 1962. Dependency in married alcoholics. *Quarterly Journal of Studies on Alcohol*. Vol. *23*: 590-609.
Lewis, M. L. 1954. The initial contact with wives of alcoholics. *Social Casework*. Vol. *35*: 8-14.
Lisansky, E. S. 1957. Alcoholism in women; social and psychological concomitants. *Quarterly Journal of Studies on Alcohol*. Vol. *18*: 588-623.
Makepeace, J. M. 1981. Courtship violence among college students. *Family Relations*. Vol. *30*, 97-102.
Makepeace, J. M. 1983. Life events stress and courtship violence. *Family Relations*. Vol. *32*, 101-109.
Malatesta, V. J., Pollack, R. H., Wilbanks, W. A., & Adams, H. E. 1979. Alcohol

effects on the orgasmic-ejaculatory response in human males. *The Journal of Sex Research.* Vol. *15*: 101-107.
McClelland, D. C., Davis, W. N., Kalin, R., & Wanner, E. 1972. *The Drinking Man.* New York: Plenum Press.
Mitchell, H. E. 1959. The interrelatedness of alcoholism and marital conflict. *American Journal of Orthopsychiatry.* Vol. *29*: 547-559.
Murphy, J. 1984. *Date abuse and forced intercourse among college students.* Paper presented at the Annual Meeting of the Midwest Sociological Society, Chicago, IL, April 18-21.
Nohre, S. 1987. Toward developing a healthy sexual lifestyle post chemical dependency treatment. *Journal of Chemical Dependency Treatment.* Vol. 1.
Paolino, T. J. & McCrady, B. A. 1977. *The Alcoholic Marriage: Alternative Perspectives.* New York: Grune & Stratton.
Paolino, T. J., McCrady, B., Diamond, S., & Diamond, R. 1976. Psychological disturbances in spouses of alcoholics: An empirical assessment. *Journal of Studies on Alcohol.* Vol. *37*: 1600-1608.
Paredes, A. 1973. Marital-sexual factors in alcoholism. *Medical Aspects of Human Sexuality.* April: 98-114.
Powell, B. J., Viamontes, J. A., & Brown, C. S. 1974. Alcohol effects on the sexual potency of alcoholic and non-alcoholic males. *Sexuality.* Vol. 10: 78-80.
Price, G. M. 1945. A study of the wives of twenty alcoholics. *Quarterly Journal of Studies on Alcohol.* Vol. *5*: 620-627.
Rae, R. B. & Drewery, J. 1972. Interpersonal patterns in alcoholic marriages. *British Journal of Psychiatry.* Vol. *120*: 615-621.
Renshaw, D. C. 1978. Impotence—Some causes and cures. *American Family Physician.* Vol. *17*: 143-146.
Roy, M. 1977. *A psychosociological study of domestic violence.* New York: Van Nostrand Reinhold. A research project probing a cross-section of battered women.
Rubin, H. B. & Henson, D. E. 1976. Effects of alcohol on male sexual responding. *Psychopharmacology.* Vol. *47*: 123-134.
Sandmaier, M. 1980. *The Invisible Alcoholics: Women and Alcohol Abuse in America.* New York: McGraw-Hill.
Schaefer, S. and Evans, S. 1987. Women, sexuality and the process of recovery. *Journal of Chemical Dependency Treatment.* Vol. *1.*
Schaefer, S., Evans, S. & Coleman, E. 1987. Sexual orientation considerations in chemical dependency treatment. *Journal of Chemical Dependency Treatment.* Vol. *1.*
Schuckit, M. 1972. Sexual disturbance in the woman alcoholic. *Medical Aspects of Human Sexuality.* Vol. 6: 44, 48-49, 53, 57, 60-61, 65.
Scott, P. D. Battered wives. 1974. *British Journal of Psychiatry.* Vol. *125*: 433-441.
Smalley, S. and Coleman, E. 1987. Treating intimacy dysfunctions in dyadic relationships among chemically dependent and codependent relationships. *Journal of Chemical Dependency Treatment.* Vol. *1.*
Smith, J. W., Lemere, F., & Dunn, R. B. 1972. Impotence in alcoholism. *Northwest Medicine.* Vol. *71*: 523-524.
Story, N. L. 1974. Sexual dysfunction resulting from drug side effects. *The Journal of Sex Research.* Vol. *10*: 132-149.
Strauss, M. 1979. Family patterns and child abuse in a nationally representative sample. *Child Abuse and Neglect.* Vol. *3*: 213-225.
Van Thiel, D. H. & Lester, R. 1976. Sex and alcohol: A second peek. *The New England Journal of Medicine.* Vol. *295*: 835-836.

Whalen, T. 1953. Wives of alcoholics: four types observed in a family service agency. *Quarterly Journal of Studies on Alcohol.* Vol. *14*: 632-641.

Wieland, W. F. & Yunger, M. 1970. *Sexual effects and side effects of heroin and methadone.* In Proceedings, Third National Conference on Methadone Treatment, New York. Washington, DC: U. S. Government Printing Office.

Wilsnack, S. C. 1976. The impact of sex roles on women's alcohol use and abuse in M. Greenblatt and M. A. Schuckit (Eds.) *Alcoholism Problems in Men and Women.* New York: Grune and Stratton.

Wilson, G. T. 1977. Alcohol and human sexual behavior. *Behavior, Research and Therapy.* Vol. *15*: 239-252.

Wilson, G. T. & Lawson, D. M. 1976a. Expectancies, alcohol and sexual arousal in male social drinkers. *Journal of Abnormal Psychology.* Vol. *85*: 587-594.

Wilson, G. T. & Lawson, D. M. 1976b. The effects of alcohol on sexual arousal in women. *Journal of Abnormal Psychology.* Vol. *85*: 489-497.

Shame, Intimacy, and Sexuality

Jeffrey A. Brown, MSE

SUMMARY. This paper examines the interrelationship between shame and problems with intimacy and sexuality. It posits the view that these problems are the manifestations primarily of difficulties in identification and differentiation in the developmental process and of the influence of culture and religion. The author recommends that intervention focus on the six developmental tasks proposed by Kaufman (1980) and concludes that treatment will succeed to the extent that interpersonal bridging, balance of identification/differentiation, and transference occur in the therapeutic relationship.

Until recently, the significance of shame has been largely ignored in the literature and offices of psychiatrists, psychologists, and psychotherapists. Shame has emerged as a missing piece in the understanding of addiction, co-dependency, sexual abuse, intimacy dysfunctions, and sexual difficulties.

Chemical dependency practitioners are beginning to view shame as one of the underlying elements in addictive behaviors. There is a growing consensus that difficulties with sexuality and intimacy are associated with dependencies. For example, victims of abuse often report that the initial abuse of chemicals was used to reduce or numb feelings of shame, rage, and hurt. Problems with intimacy in chemically dependent families are well documented (Coleman, 1983).

Shame has been defined variously as "a wound to one's self-

Jeffrey A. Brown holds a Master's Degree in Counseling Psychology and is a Licensed Psychologist. He works at the Program in Human Sexuality, Department of Family Practice and Community Health, Medical School, University of Minnesota and Southwest Family Services, P.A. Requests for reprints can be sent to the author at the Program in Human Sexuality, 2630 University Ave. S.E., Minneapolis, MN 55414.

© 1987 by The Haworth Press, Inc. All rights reserved.

esteem, a painful feeling or sense of degradation excited by the consciousness of having done something unworthy of one's previous idea of one's own excellence" (Lynd, 1961, p. 24), as "an impulse to bury one's face, or to sink, right then and there, into the ground" (Erikson, 1963, p. 252), and as a "sickness of the soul" (Kaufman, 1980, p. 13). Shame implies a total failure of self. Guilt, though commonly used interchangeably with shame, implies a transgression of a specific law, rule, or personal standard. It is not a failure of self.

FORMATION OF SHAME

Many developmental theories conceptualize shame as an indicator of disruption in the process of identification and differentiation (Kaufman, 1980; Kegan, 1982; Miller, A., 1981; Miller, S., 1985). The identity of the human being grows out of an evolving sense of belonging, wholeness, and mutuality, as well as a sense of separateness and individuality. From the safety of identification with the parental figures, the child begins to explore and develop his or her own needs, feelings, thoughts, beliefs, and values (see Figure 1).

In a shame-based family system, this process is interfered with in some way. The essential feature of this early interference is that the child is forced to disassociate from aspects of her or his emerging individuality and to over-identify with the parental figure. In order to satisfy needs to belong, to feel whole, and to feel

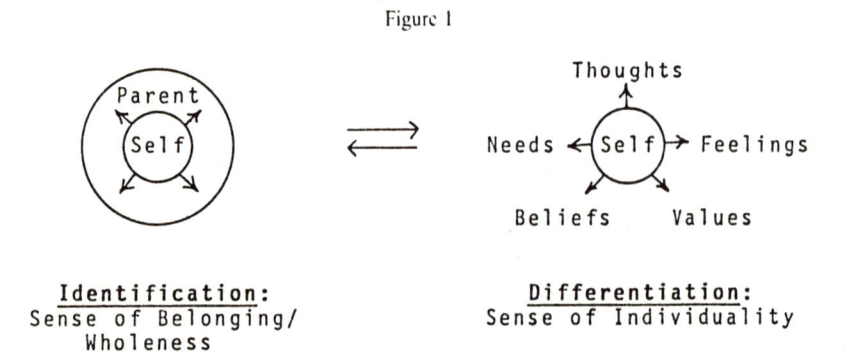

Figure 1

Identification:
Sense of Belonging/
Wholeness

Differentiation:
Sense of Individuality

a part of something larger, the child must substitute, throw away, and disengage aspects of self. These parents are individuals who seek, through their children, gratification of their own needs for security, attention, and admiration (Miller, A., 1981).

This interference apparently can occur very early, and often it "begins around the time a child can be shamed through failure/disgrace messages to move his or her bowels successfully on the potty, eat food without spilling it, sit still, and be good" (Friesen, 1979, p. 43). Erikson (1963) suggests that the development of an identity characterized by "shame and doubt" is an early phenomenon formed from a "loss of self-control and foreign over-control" (p. 254). While acknowledging that the origins of shame can occur at any point in the cycle, Kaufman (1980) suggests that shame is often first induced pre-verbally in the very young child. In her description of the creation of narcissistic disorders, Alice Miller (1981) appears to conclude that shame is a product of early childhood misadaptation. Kopp (1980) explains that the formation of a "'compliant, false self' is completed by the end of the third year of a child's life" (p. 15).

Kegan (1982) speculates that the identification/differentiation process is one that evolves throughout an individual's lifetime. Shame can occur at the crossroads of any of six stages from early childhood through the adult years. Shame has been viewed as a "developmental backslide" (Kegan, 1982) that indicates a retrospection to an earlier developmental point. Viewed in this way, various adult dysfunctions and sexual problems may not be the consequence of early developmental failure at age two or three, but of some later difficulty. Over-identification with parent and under-differentiation of the self remain the dilemma, but it is reflected in advanced expressions of the self's continuing evolution. Additionally, the parental figure is now primarily internalized or represented in the institutions of society.

FORMATION OF SHAME-RELATED INTIMACY DYSFUNCTION

Since shame initially occurs out of the interplay with another person (usually the parent), it is fundamentally an interpersonal problem. There has been some failure in relating to another and to the self. Kaufman (1980) refers to this process as the breaking of an "interpersonal bridge." In the simplest sense, the bridge is formed between two people out of a repeated interchange of understanding, trust, and security from which a mutuality and feeling of certainty emerge. The bridge is broken when someone betrays the understanding, trust, and security. A feeling of being made vulnerable and exposed eventuates in self-mistrust, doubt, and shame.

In the identification/differentiation process, the interpersonal bridge is broken whenever the individual is somehow coerced to substitute the other's identity for their own, or whenever significant aspects of the individual are repudiated directly or indirectly. The shame that erupts is the outcome of the individual's perceived or actual inability to form an intimate attachment in which his or her own needs, feelings, thoughts, beliefs, and values are accepted by the other. In summary, a pattern occurs that precludes a balance of identification and differentiation that appears to be necessary for intimate relationships (Coleman & Colgan, 1986).

Several theorists have identified factors during a child's development that seem to contribute to this failure of balanced identification/differentiation and the consequent intimacy dysfunction. One of the factors identified by Friesen (1979) is the reduction of family members from significant others to "Others" (p. 49). In these systems, members become "bound" as extensions of the parents or objects for the parent's own expression. Accordingly, no real relationship exists; "trust, intimacy, love, and pain are distanced and lost" (Friesen, 1979, p. 49).

Stierlin and Ravenscroft (1972) suggest that a family member may be bound to a parent in one of three ways. On one level the parent can infantalize and spoil the child into a compliancy and submissiveness sufficient to prevent the child from differentiating. On a second level, the parent can bind the child by interfering with the ability to express independent needs, motives, and goals. On a third level, the parent can bind the child through massive conscious and unconscious uses of loyalty demands and shaming. Depending on the mode of binding, one can expect difficulties in handling conflicts, articulating feelings, needs, and wants, or in resolving feelings of "breakaway guilt" (p. 301).

A second factor appears to be the exclusion or limitation of certain emotions. Stierlin (1974) speculates that these systems allow expressions of angry and hostile feelings, but disallow tender and loving ones. Kaufman (1980, p. 4) describes "affect shame binds" as the way in which any emotions can become associated with shame and eventually become excluded from intimate interaction. Initially, the child's response to particular emotions are either directly or indirectly shamed. This process eventually becomes internalized; shame becomes sufficiently associated with the primary emotion so that it serves as a defense against that emotion. In the end, certain feelings are excluded from expression, sometimes to the extent that the individual is totally unaware of them.

A third factor is that of internal versus external locus of control. The concept refers to a continuum from exclusive external reference of behaviors to exclusive internal reference of behaviors (Engler, 1985, p. 420). Externally referenced individuals would consider their behavior to be out of their control and subject to the impact of other people, situations, and luck. Internally referenced individuals would consider their behavior to be the result of their choices which they are responsible for.

Developmentally, one would expect that the child would increase in internality as he or she grows. Family conditions that are warm and supportive and that encourage independence and responsibility assure movement toward internality (Lefcourt, 1976). On the other hand, family reactions such as anger, rejection, threats of abandonment, rigid rules, and use of punishment as humiliation would assure movement toward externality. The externality in the shame-based system prevents the child from developing a sense of responsible self in the world by interfering with opportunities to test out logical consequences, try behaviors, and make mistakes.

FORMATION OF SEXUAL SHAME

Many of the foundations of sexual shame are the same as those of shame related intimacy dysfunctions. However, some types of sexual shame have specific, identifiable origins. Among these are: poor body image, some instances of sexual dysfunction and lack of sexual desire, discomfort with masturbation, and sexual identity dysphoria.

Kaufman's (1980, p. 49) conceptualization of "drive shame binds" is helpful in understanding the formation of sexual shame. According to this model, certain drives, including sexuality, become associated with shame in the same manner as affect shame binds. That is, sexual behaviors and expressions are repeatedly paired with shaming, parental responses until the shame becomes internalized and functions as a defense. However, this model does not account for the more destructive or inappropriate sexual behaviors. Perhaps in these cases, the behavior is an expression of shame and can no longer be defended against (see Figure 2).

The formation of the more common expressions of sexual shame can be attributed to family dynamics, lack of information, religion, and early childhood experiences (Fischer, 1986). This shame may have originated previously out of cultural or religious experiences or from some family secret. Consequently, specific rules and expectations about referring to sex, touching, and appropriate behavior were developed.

In many families, shame about sexuality is a multi-generalization issue. Most children acquire a sense of appropriate touch before they are able to speak. In changing the baby's diaper, for example, parents may react differently or touch differently when

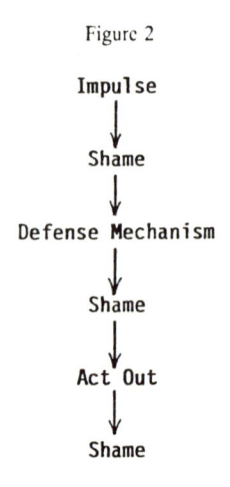

Figure 2

Impulse
↓
Shame
↓
Defense Mechanism
↓
Shame
↓
Act Out
↓
Shame

they near the genital area. From observing how the parents touch them and each other, and later from the ways they are allowed to touch others, children develop rules of touch and perceptions of the acceptability of their bodies. Language about sex may be absent, communicated only through euphemisms, or referred to in anger or distaste. In all cases, shame is the underlying content. Certain family rules, frequently revolving around self-pleasuring, gender appropriate behavior, and general display or expression of affection, often serve to shame what are normal experiences and reflections of individual differences.

Although the general level of information available about sex has increased dramatically in the last twenty years, many parents have done little to provide accurate information on a continuing basis to their developing children. This lack of information communicates a basic discomfort with, and shame about the subject, and it interferes with the child's reality testing about sexuality. Consequently, numerous normal sexual experiences are conceived of as something bad, dirty, or unnatural.

The impact of religion on sexual shame has been widely discussed since the sexual revolution (Nelson, 1978). The concept of sex as sin has been supported with specific messages about masturbation, homosexuality, and any other sexual activity other than "missionary position" activity. When normal sexual expressions come in conflict with this concept of sin and other specific messages, the opportunities for shame arise.

In other cases, sexual shame is an expression of variance between individual beliefs and behaviors and the church's conception of male/female roles, mind and body separation, and the purposes of sex. Religious and cultural sanctions have reinforced male roles of independence, self-assertion, personal achievement, and performance (differentiation) and female roles of fusion, dependence, and emotionality (identification) (Kegan, 1982, p. 208). These role expectations limit natural expression of sexuality and require that the individual dissociate from aspects of self. The view of mind as separate from body creates a chasm between feelings and self, body and identity, and a conflict with the sensuous aspects of self. New viewpoints embracing the pleasurable aspects of self, as opposed to the procreative aspect, have generated dissonance and shame for many, especially in regard to masturbation, homosexuality, and premarital sex. In some cases, shame arises out of a more general sense that the individual's sexuality is at odds with her or his spirituality; as such, it is an ethical problem that extends beyond psychological concepts alone.

Early childhood experiences can become coupled with shame in two ways. Some experiences, notably physical, sexual, or emotional abuse, almost implicitly create conditions of shame. Other experiences, which are common and associated with normal development and experimentation, can be shame producing if poorly handled. Physical, sexual, or emotional abuse of the child interferes with the process of identification/differentiation in significant ways. When the abuser is the parent or important adult/caregiver, the child must choose the impossible: to identify with the abusing person, or to detach from him/her. Safety, which is the hallmark for the development of healthy differentiation, has been seriously jeopardized as well. At its deepest level, this shame is an expression of the bind that forces the child to abandon aspects of himself or herself in order to survive. Common sexual experiences in a child's life, such as masturbation, sex play, and same-sex exploration, can be as shame producing when the parent overreacts or misperceives the meaning of the behavior.

INTIMACY AND SHAME IN ADULTHOOD

Interpersonal problems experienced by the majority of shame-based adults will be the result of over-identification and under-differentiation in the relationship. When both partners are under-differentiated, individual goal activity and autonomy are absent, and patterns of interaction are rigid. The two individuals are essentially fused into each other and the continuing struggle "to determine whose stand will represent their relationship" will be common (Berezowsky, 1976, p. 99). Since this interaction is basically a replication of an earlier intimacy dysfunction, one would also expect parallel problems with objectification, exclusion of certain emotions, and an external locus of control. An overriding fear of abandonment if the individual expresses too much separateness in identity, and engulfment if the individual becomes too fused, can also be expected.

It is not coincidental that these types of relationships are also described as co-dependent or dependent. The underlying expectation is that one individual will find completion of self in the other. The individual is transferring upon his or her partner all of the unmet needs for identification and differentiation that he or she failed to get at some developmental point. The tragedy, of course, is that this is an impossible feat and one that often ends in bitterness and resentment toward the person who is unable to complete the other.

Generally, when one partner is over-differentiated, and the other over-identified, the male will typically be over-differentiated and the female typically over-identified. The evolution of intimacy dysfunction and shame will centralize around each individual's capacity to sufficiently embrace the other aspect. Thus, the male's shame will characteristically revolve around his inability to provide sensitivity, support, warmth, and inclusion. The female's shame will revolve around her inability to be self-directed, autonomous, and assertive (Kegan, 1982, p. 210). Consequently, the male's fear is engulfment; the female's fear is abandonment. Fortunately, the women's movement has challenged these rigid and intimacy hampering roles, and this culture is beginning to make some adjustments.

SEXUAL SHAME IN ADULTHOOD

Sexual shame in adulthood often solidifies around a specific issue, such as sexual identity or sex role gender dysphoria, sexual offending behavior, continued victim experiences, lack of sexual desire, sexual dysfunction, and shame about masturbation.

For example, the sexual identity dysphoric male homosexual is an individual whose emerging sexuality as an aspect of differentiation/identification has been interfered with. He is struggling to embrace his sexuality despite societal and religious attitudes, stereotypes, negative role models, and fear of loss. To accept his homosexuality is to differentiate in an unacceptable way. To reject his homosexuality is to deny his identity.

Victims of sexual abuse often report engaging in extremes of sexual behavior ranging from a total lack of sexual interest to destructively promiscuous behavior. In either extreme, the task is to reclaim aspects of self and development. Often, this involves accepting sexual feelings and sensations that were previously associated with the abuse, and consequently thrown away.

Lack of sexual desire, sexual dysfunction, and shame about masturbation can partially be manifestations of an inability to accept the personal sexual self. In these types of sexual shame, the earlier, natural sexuality and sensuality of the child has been marred by a lack of trust, over-constriction, and poor body image. The individual is unable to trust that his or her sexual sensations, feelings, and sensuousness are natural expressions. His or her shame constricts the arena of sexuality to a very limited, almost nonexistent sphere. Poor body image is often a coexisting element. This may be a reflection of an inaccurate perception of body, mistaken views of the body as something dirty or unacceptable, or unreasonable appearance expectations.

OVERVIEW OF INTERVENTION/TREATMENT

Intervention can occur at a variety of levels. It may involve giving permission for the individual to explore, think about, or express various aspects of shame. The importance of accurate information giving cannot be understated, especially in the area of sexuality. Often, misconceptions, myths, fears, and beliefs can be ameliorated with reliable, current data. People can often benefit from specific suggestions provided by self-help groups, books, and workshops.

Intervention on the level of intensive therapy should operate out of certain assumptions, no matter which specific modality or approach is utilized. The clinician's role is not to rid this client of his or her shame. Shame is not pathological. At appropriate levels, shame can assist in spiritual and emotional growth and function as a brake to certain behaviors. Conceptualizing shame as a stepping stone or as a signal of some "developmental backslide" (Kegan, 1982, p. 216) will help in removing the pathological element. Since the development of shame is understood in the context of identity formation and interpersonal interactions, the overall therapy should be directed towards advancing growth in these areas. Specifically, focus on issues involving differentiation/identification and interpersonal bridging would be important. An eclectic approach that looks at emotions, beliefs systems, behaviors, and the underlying content, is probably the most effective, since shame appears to function at these levels (see Figure 3).

Intervention by the chemical dependency practitioner can focus on identity formation and interpersonal functioning as part of the primary treatment. While intervention for most shame-based individuals needs to occur over a longer period than the relatively brief and intensive treatment characterized by most chemical dependency approaches, the chemical dependency treatment can be a forum for: (1) supporting initial disclosure of shame issues, (2) beginning interpersonal bridging, (3) assessing problems with sexuality and intimacy, and (4) making appropriate aftercare referrals. The practitioner's approach should be supportive and non-shaming and should model appropriate expressions of shame. Confrontation that is factual, nonjudgemental, and respectful will reduce the eliciting of shame responses. Group treatment that focuses on the interpersonal bridging of various members will serve as a model for expression of shameful feelings, thoughts, and behaviors.

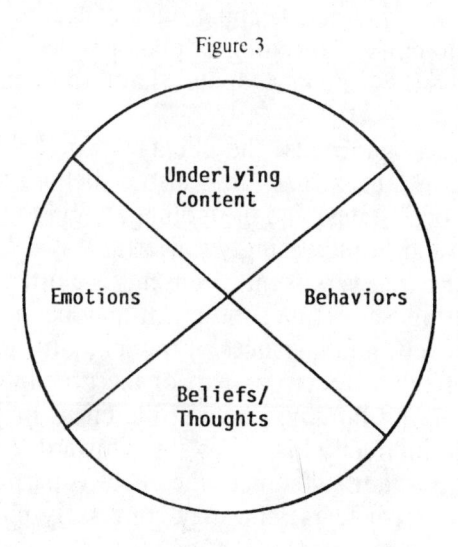

Figure 3

A TREATMENT MODEL

Kaufman (1980, pp. 152-159), suggests that the healing of shame involves six developmental tasks: differential owning capacity, reintegrating of self, developing internal security, self-nurturance, self-affirmation, and attaining a separate identity.

Differentiated owning capacity and reintegrating of self (Kaufman, 1980, pp. 156-158, 153-154) includes separating, owning, and reintegrating emotions, beliefs, needs, wants, and aspects of self that had been discarded. The essential element in assisting in the development of differential owning capacity and reintegration of self is the therapeutic relationship. This relationship will be effective to the extent that interpersonal bridging, balance of identification/differentiation, and transference occur. The therapist is essentially re-parenting the client and in so doing is providing an opportunity for healthier identification and differentiation. A task of this sort is difficult, and it requires that the clinician be trustworthy and honest and that he or she provide ample amounts of security.

In the early phases of this process, the therapist's task is to assist the client in clarifying beliefs, feelings, needs, and thoughts and in identifying shameful material. Initially, the client may have a difficult time in separating and owning these aspects of self. Keeping a journal, keeping track of feelings, dialoguing with "the little child," bringing in photographs of self, and returning to previous "memory spots" have all been found to be helpful.

As this process proceeds, the client will probably remember more shaming instances. They may also be better able to identify specific emotional states, and in so doing, begin to relate to them more directly and in increasingly powerful ways. Letters to self and parents or caregivers (sent or unsent) are often important at this point. At this same time, the client may begin to grieve for lost aspects of self, and instances of trauma, hurt, pain, sadness, and rage are likely to occur as part of the grieving process. As part of the working-through process, the client may transfer either directly or indirectly his or her anger toward the parent upon the therapist. In the transference, the client is particularly sensitive to abandonment fears, and may conversely make efforts to abandon the therapist first. As the anger and sadness subside, a deep sense of loss of direction and disconnectedness may follow. This is a critical point in therapy, since the client is most vulnerable to returning to old shame based expressions of identity as a reaction to feeling without an identity.

Conjointly with this process, the clinician will need to focus on developing internal security. Specific defenses should be identified and the underlying material revealed. This is a delicate process, since any confrontation can be easily viewed as additional shaming. The best approach may be to utilize an objective stance, commenting on material that appears to be defended against, and providing assignments in learning about the nature of defensive situations, and journalizing personal uses of them.

Following the completion of the grieving process, the client should be assisted in developing self-affirming and self-nurturing behavior. Specific negative behavior patterns, destructive self talk, and useless belief systems can be identified as the first step of this process. Use of specific goals, contracts, and positive affirmations will help counteract non-affirming and non-nurturing elements.

In encouraging the client to attain a separate identity, the clinician should emphasize the process of interpersonal bridging. Therapy groups may be a transition to interpersonal bridging in the larger society. Teaching specific skills in assertiveness, communication, and parenting may be helpful. The therapist may also consider including significant others in the therapy process at this point. Spirituality can be introduced as a concept and various books, support groups, and spiritual figures can be recommended.

Intervention with specific sexual or intimacy issues requires specialized techniques and competency that are beyond the scope of this chapter. Referral to a marital or sexual therapist is the most appropriate intervention in these cases.

REFERENCES

Berezowsky, J. (1976). Intimacy, individuation, and marriage. *Canadian Counselor*, *13*(2), 98-101.
Coleman, E. (1983). Sexuality and the alcoholic family: Effects of chemical depen-

dence and codependence upon individual family members. In *Alcoholism: Analysis of a world-wide problem*, P. Golding (Ed.) Lancaster, England: MTP Press Limited.

Coleman, E. & Colgan, P. (1986). Boundary inadequacy in chemically dependent families. *Journal of Psychoactive Drugs. 18*, 21-30.

Engler, B. (1985). *Personality theories*. Boston: Houghton Mifflin.

Erikson, E. (1963). *Childhood and society* (2nd ed.). New York: Norton.

Fischer, B. (1985, December). *Sexuality and shame*. Symposium conducted at The Program in Human Sexuality, University of Minnesota, Minneapolis, MN.

Friesen, V. (1979). On shame and the family. *Family Therapy, 6*(1), 39-57.

Kaufman, G. (1980). *Shame: The power of caring*. Cambridge: Shenkman.

Kegan, R. (1982). *The evolving self: Problems and processes in human development*. Cambridge: Howard University Press.

Kopp, S. (1980). *Mirror, mask and shadow: The risks and rewards of self acceptance*. New York: MacMillan.

Lefcourt, H. (1976). *Locus of control: Current trends in theory and research*. Hillsdale, NJ: Erlbaum.

Lynd, H. (1985). *On shame and the search for identity*. New York: Harcourt, Brace, and World.

Miller, A. (1981). *The drama of the gifted child: How narcissistic parents form and deform the emotional lives of their talented children*. New York: Basic Books.

Miller, S. (1985). *The shame experience*. Hillsdale, NJ: Analytic Press.

Nelson, J. (1978). *Embodiment: An approach to sexuality and Christian theology*. Minneapolis: Augsburg Publishing House.

Stierlin, H. (1974). Shame and guilt in family relations: Theoretical and clinical aspects. *Archives of General Psychiatry, 30*, 381-389.

Stierlin, H., & Ravenscroft, K. (1972). Varieties of adolescent 'separation conflicts.' *British Journal of Medical Psychiatry, 45*, 299-313.

Assessment of Boundary Inadequacy in Chemically Dependent Individuals and Families

Philip Colgan, MA

SUMMARY. Interpersonal boundary inadequacy has been highly correlated with chemical dependence in both individuals and families. Accurate assessment of patterns of boundary inadequacy appears integral to the successful recovery process of chemically dependent people. This paper presents a conceptual approach for skillful assessment of boundary inadequacy.

Boundary inadequacy has been defined as a pattern of ambiguous, overly rigid, or invasive boundaries related to physical or psychological space. These patterns have been found to be highly correlated with chemically dependent individuals and families (Coleman and Colgan, 1986).

Clinicians (e.g., Neilsen, 1984; Schaefer and Evans, 1984) have referred to the necessity for adequate assessment and treatment of boundary inadequacy as an integral part of recovery for chemically dependent individuals and families.

Skillful assessment of boundary inadequacy patterns involves (1) a thorough and integrated professional knowledge of boundary inadequacies; (2) a thorough and integrated personal knowledge of one's own history with or potential for boundary inade-

---

Philip Colgan is in private practice as a licensed psychologist in Minneapolis, MN. He has a clinical appointment at the Program in Human Sexuality, Department of Family Practice and Community Health, Medical School, University of Minnesota.

Requests for reprints can be sent to the author at the Program in Human Sexuality, 2630 University Avenue, S.E., Minneapolis, MN 55414.

The author would like to especially thank Richard Kott, Ann Stefanson, and Geol Weirs for their contributions.

quacy; (3) a disciplined respect for individual differences; and (4) practice, conducted in consultation with other professionals in the field. This paper will address these four components of assessment.

BOUNDARY INADEQUACY

Coleman and Colgan (1986) provide descriptions of three observed patterns of boundary inadequacy: ambiguous, overly rigid, and invasive. Ambiguous boundary inadequacy involves a pattern of double messages exchanged within the relationship. The double messages (e.g., "I'm going to kill myself, but don't tell anybody") create an atmosphere of tension wherein the recipient of the communication can never be sure what can be believed. The inability of the communicator to send clear messages lays the groundwork for the cycle of ambiguity to begin.

Overly rigid boundary inadequacy is characterized by patterns of behavior wherein smooth and efficient functioning is a priority over being responsive and adaptable. Adherence to a preset code of behavior, regardless of intervening situational variables, leads to patterns of interaction wherein roles are played and rules followed. This gives the appearance of interdependence. But in reality, all actors within the system are dependent on the system, with its rules and roles. They do not depend on one another as people who can be responsive.

Invasive boundary inadequacy involves patterns of behavior wherein an imbalance of power is used to objectify people. The clear examples of sexual and physical abuse illustrate the rule governing this dynamic: all but the rights of the actor are nullified. Other people become objects for the actor to use in satisfying all needs.

These three types of boundary inadequacy can be expressed through physical or psychological interactions. For example:

Ambiguous:

Physical: a friendship hug which includes a body caress.
Psychological: "Let's go on a picnic sometime."

Overly Rigid:

>Physical: Hugs are exchanged only at airports.
>Psychological: "What will the neighbors think?"

Invasive:

>Physical: Sexual and/or physical abuse.
>Psychological: Prying or shaming.

These are offered only as examples to illustrate the diversity — from subtle to blatant — involved in boundary inadequacy. All three types of patterns of boundary inadequacy — ambiguous, overly rigid, and invasive — share elements of (a) confusion between dependence and caring; (b) disrespect for or ignorance of the relationship between interdependence and individual differences; and (c) confusion between independence and personal power. These elements may appear as themes emerging from the assessment.

DEPENDENCE AND CARING

Boundary inadequacy can result when dependence and caring are confused. To help clients distinguish the two, I refer to dependence in terms of action and caring in terms of emotion. In its most basic state, dependence refers to the trust we place in ourselves and others to meet our expectations through action. For example, I depend on the Post Office to deliver my mail. Dependence, however, is not necessarily connected with caring. I may or may not have a close personal relationship with the letter carrier.

Caring, on the other hand, emphasizes an emotional connection over action. In this regard, caring refers to an emotional state of involvement with self and others. For example, if my friend in St. Louis writes me that she is unhappy with her job, this influences my well-being. Such influence, however, may or may not involve action: I am not expected to fly to St. Louis to right what is wrong.

Dependence and caring are often interwoven in close relationships. The closer the relationship, the more interwoven. Confusion results when the two become not merely intertwined, but inseparable. How this happens in pair bonding is easily seen: two people who choose to share their lives soon develop patterns of interaction that are repetitive in nature. Repetition becomes habit. Soon the habits have more weight than the choices. The dependability of habit becomes a substitute for the freedom of choice.

Choice is integral to healthy expressions of dependency and caring (Colgan, 1987). Lack of choice, however, leads to blurred interpersonal boundaries. Boundary inadequacy is then a likely outcome.

The oft-cited "If I care about you, then I won't burden you with my troubles" reveals the depth of confusion seen in some chemically dependent families. "My troubles" often refers to unexpressed emotions of anger and frustration directed toward the behaviorally undependable and emotionally unpredictable partner. "Martyr" like behavior, passive-aggressive behavior, withdrawal through addiction, and other dysfunctional communication systems become operative as the resentment toward the "loved one" builds.

Double messages can be seen as attempts to cope with the internal dissonance: to both be true to oneself, and to protect the other from the mounting rage. The desire for freedom of choice is viewed as incongruent with the obligations of dependability. An inability to distinguish the two is a form of boundary ambiguity. This internal boundary inadequacy then drives a cycle of chaos and boredom in the relationship.

INTERDEPENDENCE AND INDIVIDUAL DIFFERENCES

Interdependence in optimal interpersonal functioning is a desired goal wherein people are able to mutually rely on one another for both smooth daily functioning (such as a division of chores) and for give and take in emotional nurturing (such as being the "strong one" in times of crisis). This is best achieved when individual differences are respected; that is, when the various talents, skills, and communication styles of the partners are valued for their unique contribution to the interaction.

When individual differences are not understood, accepted, and valued, interdependence is lost in a battle for control of the relationship. Each person tries to mold the other into someone more acceptable. Attempts to change another's behavior, thoughts, and/or feelings, are, of course, eventually met with resistance and resentment. Interdependence crumbles to "leave me alone" coupled with "I'll do my thing, you do yours."

INDEPENDENCE AND PERSONAL POWER

In chemically dependent families, emotional isolation is frequently experienced within emotionally enmeshed family systems. Recognizing the need for disengaging from the enmeshed system, but denying the emotional pain of this, families or family members may act in ways they label "independent." When, however, independence is defined in this reactive way ("I don't need you; I can do it by myself"), the inherent, if subtle, disappointment in having to go it alone is sometimes made palatable by reframing the isolation as personal power.

When taken to extremes, this approach to life and relationships takes on a righteous and defiant quality which lays the groundwork for boundary inadequacy through disrespect of others' and one's own needs. Physical and psychological needs, if recognized at all, are frequently flattened under the steam-rolling will to power. As Finkelhor (1981) has noted, such persons act to compensate for their perceived lack of or loss of power.

Those with adequate boundaries respect the impact their behavior may have on others. Their personal power, that of true independence, is not achieved by sacrificing another's needs, but rather is undertaken with assertive respect for individuality. Power becomes defined as power over oneself, not over others.

Personally powerful people influence others by engendering respect and emulation. They encourage others to develop their own personal power, and so have no need for power over others. Having power over others would become an unpalatable boundary violation.

THE ASSESSMENT

An assessment of boundary inadequacy can be skillfully completed through an examination of psychological and physical boundaries in both the current living situation, and in the family of origin. Because patterns of boundary inadequacy are intergenerationally transmitted, the client's early learning provides the basis for current boundary inadequacy. For this reason, the outline (see Figure 1) is a suggested, not exhaustive, review of possible avenues of inquiry regarding the family of origin.

Six areas of discussion give adequate data to assess the degree and types of boundary inadequacy experienced by the individual or family. Taken as a whole, data from the six areas will give the clinician an understanding of how the client views physical and psychological boundaries. These data may show patterns in how the client perceives dependence and caring, interdependence and individual differences, and independence and personal power.

Figure 1.

BOUNDARIES ASSESSMENT

1. Person's conception of boundaries

   —describe current sources of satisfaction for boundary needs
   —describe current concerns about boundary issues

2. Communication

   —self disclosure
   —interaction for emotional give and take
   —problem solving
   —expression of feelings

3. Values

   —behavior considered appropriate for whom
   —discrepancies between what was said and what was done
   —sexual behavior considered appropriate for children
   —sensual behavior considered appropriate for children

Figure 1 continued

4. Sex Roles

   — power balance
   — decision making processes
   — achievement encouragement — sex differences
   — respect for individual differences — sex differences

5. Touch

   — expressions of affection
   — disciplining of children
   — meaning of touch to each person
   — meeting needs to touch and be touched

6. Privacy

   — conventions about nudity
   — rules about doors (open, shut, knock?)
   — sleeping arrangements
   — bathing and dressing patterns

PSYCHOLOGICAL BOUNDARY ISSUES

Those aspects of the assessment concerning primarily psychological issues include the person's conception of boundaries, their communication patterns, their values or philosophy of living, and their beliefs about sex roles.

Current understanding of boundaries — To establish a common language, it is usually helpful to directly ask the person how they understand boundaries: their definitions, importance in family relationships, role in establishing codes of behavior, and function in childrearing. This common language will provide the basis for the rest of the assessment.

Communication — It is widely recognized that poor communication characterizes most chemically dependent individuals and families. Boundary inadequacy in communication patterns is often the culmination of years of lies, denial, broken promises, etc. Several patterns may occur: the ambiguous pattern is seen in rationalizations, double messages, a lack of problem solving skills, and indirect self-disclosure. The rigid pattern is characterized by communication which is restricted to problem solving, with practical solutions preferred over emotional self-disclosure or responsiveness. The invasive pattern is seen when only one person does the "communicating," and only about his/her demands.

The goal in assessing communication patterns is to discover where lines of communication were open, and where they were closed. This will give some evidence of how patterns of interpersonal trust were learned and what patterns have been practiced.

Values — Among chemically dependent families, as in other families, values are communicated in subtle, yet easily recalled statements or events which reveal the philosophy of life as preached, or practiced, by the parent(s). Studies of addicted, enmeshed family systems (e.g., Johnson and Flach, 1985) have shown that children are frequently placed in a double bind: what is preached is not what is practiced. Psychological boundary inadequacy results when children are forced to make decisions for themselves (and for others) without the dependable guidance of parents.

The important variables in this portion of the assessment have to do with (1) what values were communicated? (2) what values were practiced? (3) what decisions the client made regarding his/her own life.

Sex roles — Several researchers have documented the connection between sex role stereotyping and chemical dependence. Filstead (1984) has suggested that societal norms and sex role definitions contribute to the gender differences in the development of alcoholism. Beckman (1984) has suggested that sex role stereotyping may both contribute to and create boundary inadequacies for the recovering female alcoholic.

Impressive evidence exists to suggest that many forms of boundary inadequacy (e.g., the sexual and physical abuse of children) have strong connections with sex role stereotyping. From the literature on sex roles, we know that sex role stereotyping is learned very early in life, and that it has formidable consequences in adult behavior. Examination of early learning about sex roles will give a greater understanding of the client's conceptions of boundary inadequacy regarding roles and expectations for males and females, and in their interactions.

PHYSICAL BOUNDARY ISSUES

Assessment of physical boundary issues focuses on what people learned about having both physical attachment and physical separation from others. Aspects of attachment are grouped under the category of touch. Aspects of separation are grouped under the category privacy. The behavioral aspects of touch and privacy are investigated to understand the client's personal learning about attachment and separation in close relationships.

Touch — Montagu (1971) notes that tactile experience plays a fundamentally important role in the growth and development of humans. Touch which is nurturing and accepting in childhood forms the basis of our positive contact with the world throughout life. Tactile deprivation, or more active punishing or abusive touch, appears to create an expectation that human relationships are and can be expected to be unsatisfying at best, violent at worst.

The goal of this section in the assessment is to learn about the patterns of touch experienced by the client as a child. Boundary inadequacy is revealed in three forms: the lack of warm, nurturing touch; touch which is ambiguous in nature (e.g., is it nurturing or sexual?); or touch which is invasive. While the importance of physical or sexual abuse has been clearly observed, other forms of touch inadequacy may be equally important. The clinician who is cognizant of this can be particularly useful in helping the clients recognize boundary inadequacy in touch even when overt abuse is absent.

Privacy — The need for and respect of privacy appears to be central to the development of healthy interpersonal boundaries. In this discussion, privacy refers to those aspects of physical space which, when respected, give children a sense of mastery over their environments, including their bodies. The goal of assessment here is to understand the particular ways in which clients learned to control physical separation from others, including behavioral aspects of touch, dressing, and bathing. Examples of healthy boundaries include respecting closed doors, knocking before entering, responding to requests to be left alone, and respecting the inherent exclusivity of letters, diaries, and phone conversations.

ASSESSMENT: THE ROLE OF THE CLINICIAN

Personal Preparation

In his discussion of sexuality education for the health care professional, Maddock (1975) has argued that the practitioner best serves clients by being aware of and knowledgeable about his/her personal attitudes about sexuality and sexual behavior. A parallel argument can be developed in the case of assessment of boundary inadequacy.

The most helpful clinicians will be those who have examined boundary inadequacy personally. This can be completed within or in addition to professional training. Examination of one's own history with boundary inadequacy can reveal one's potential for creating boundary inadequacy in personal and professional relationships. This self-referenced approach is healthy prevention of counselor-client boundary inadequacy. As Coleman and Schaefer (1986) have noted, counselors who meet their needs at the expense of client needs violate interpersonal boundaries in subtle ways which undermine the counselor's power, and often lead to more blatant forms of intrusion.

The clinician who is unable to set and stick to respectful limits conveys two messages to the client(s): (1) that the clinician has nothing positive to teach about boundaries and (2) that the client has no need to recognize or respect interpersonal boundaries in order to recover from chemical dependency.

Health care professionals who assess boundary inadequacy will be more skillful in offering clinical help by recognizing their own limitations in setting and observing interpersonal boundaries. For example, observing the time limits of appointments, setting limits on the amount of contact outside of treatment, and protecting one's homelife against unwanted intrusions by clients are all necessary for congruent modelling of appropriate interpersonal boundaries.

Ongoing examination of transference and counter-transference issues is a routine part of ethical practice. It is especially crucial in the assessment of boundary inadequacies. Self-examination can begin, or be repeated, using the guidelines in Figure 1. As always in matters of professional training and review, this is of course best examined and discussed with others whose boundaries can be depended upon and respected.

Professional Preparation: Respect for Individual Differences

In chemically dependent individuals and families, as in others, what is acceptable will vary from person to person. Clinicians have noted, for example, that similar experiences with touch will have very different meanings for different clients.

The experience of physical abuse serves as a good example. Researchers (e.g., Solomon, 1980) have reported the phenomenon of the physical organism becoming so accustomed to physical pain that further episodes of the same behavior become meaningless. For others, the rare occasion of physical aggression directed toward them can create lasting psychological damage.

What appears to be most salient in the accurate assessment of boundary inadequacy, both historically and in the present, is the context or personal meaning the person attaches to inadequate or adequate boundaries.

It is for this reason that the assessment has to do with reactions and responses to patterns of behavior which are personally meaningful. Over time, a specific behavior repeated in a specific context may or may not assume a private meaning for the recipient of boundary inadequacies. For many, repeated behaviors will represent a family ritual which reinforces developing concepts about what one can and should expect in human interactions (see Wolin, Bennett, and Noonan, 1979). This, of course, represents a portion of the cycle of intergenerational transmission of boundary inadequacy, as shown by Coleman and Colgan (1986).

For others, the patterns of boundary inadequacy will represent the chaotic and unpredictable nature of chemically dependent systems. For such persons and families, the specific behavior is perhaps less important than the tension expected in an unstable environment. Broken promises, unpredictable parenting (e.g., parents vacillating between being affectionate and rejecting for no apparent reason), and communication patterns which involve imperatives such as "Do as I say, not as I do!" can all create the unstable atmosphere. Expectations about life, people, and their interactions are shaped in a distorted perception of what is "normal" (Woititz, 1983).

Without other input, the person reared in such an environment will become even more confounded and perplexed when new data in the form of comparison with others occurs, either in childhood or in the formative stages of some adult relationships. The health care professional's understanding of the client's personal, emotional interpretation of life's events becomes paramount for accurate assessment of boundary inadequacy.

Assessment: Thematic Trends

The personal, emotional interpretations of life's events form life themes for clients from chemically dependent systems. These life-themes will emerge in a skillful assessment. The client's themes reveal internal evaluations about themselves and their boundaries. Independence, dependence, and interdependence are frequently seen interwoven with idiosyncratic perceptions of personal power, caring, and the inherent value of individual differences.

Overriding most themes resulting from boundary inadequacies is the decision that one is personally and irrevocably defective in a fundamental way. The perceived deficit is personalized as a theme of responsibility for the actions of others. Many (e.g., Mason and Fossum, 1986; Kaufman, 1974) have identified this internal condemnation of self as "shame."

A brief description of shame by example may be helpful. The decision of a child to blame herself for the parent's/parents' alcoholism is one example. The decision is made in isolation from data other than what the child's ego-centric frame of reference provides. Such a child is likely to interpret the parent's/parents' alcoholism as a suitable response to the child being herself—a child—with all the inadequacies and inconsistencies of learning how to be an adult. The decision forms a basis for developing boundary inadequacies which thematically recur in later human relationships of all kinds.

An assessment of shame as the result of interpersonal boundary inadequacy is best conducted in a straightforward manner which respects the right of the individual to feel ashamed, even when such a decision contradicts available evidence. Simple questions which open the door for the clients to discuss those thoughts, feelings, or behaviors they feel ashamed about are best. A direct and accepting approach communicates to clients that whatever they feel shame about can be discussed openly with a nonjudgmental listener.

A thorough discussion of shame as a life-theme will reveal some of the deepest interpersonal boundary problems clients have. The boundary inadequacy learned through growing up "shame-based" can be expressed in the adult as responsibility to see that such treatment is never visited on another. This decision will have ramifications in adult relationships when people protect others from shame by hiding or keeping secret their fears, anxieties, angers, frustrations—the "negative" emotions. Such patterns of protection clearly involve personal definitions about caring, power, and individuality which are confused with independence, interdependence, and dependence.

Another outcome has been observed in the adult children of chemically dependent parents. Smalley (1982) refers to this outcome as the "underresponsible" adult. "Once a loser, always a loser" was one client's description of himself in assessment. Having decided as a child that he was powerless to change, alter, or influence the behavior of the adults, he continued in his own adulthood to be under-responsible by avoiding any situation which required him to be assertive or accountable. His perceptions of the theme discussed above are at once predictable and individual.

Clearly, clinicians who are familiar with shame as a clinical label for a personal process of self-evaluation will serve their clients by withholding judgment or interpretation of the client's thoughts, feelings, or behavior. Idiosyncratic interpretations of independence, dependence, and interdependence are not amenable to intervention at this point. For this reason, an attitude of respect for individual differences becomes crucial for an excellent assessment.

Practice

Undertaking a skillful assessment of boundary inadequacy involves a practiced understanding of the dialogue between client and professional. Understanding the dynamics of boundary inadequacy, ranging from the overt and obvious (such as physical or sexual abuse) to the covert and subtle (such as shame), forms an essential basis for the direction of questioning. Understanding that individuals and families with similar patterns of boundaries may make different personal interpretations of those boundaries forms the basis for nonjudgmental respect of individual differences. Together with one's personal knowledge of boundary inadequacies, these bases knit together in the professional's attitudinal approach to the assessment.

The attitude is one of acceptance and interest. It is perhaps best described as curiosity, or "teach me about you." Clients, given enough room, will teach us what we as health care professionals need to know about their boundaries and their boundary inadequacies. This personalized knowledge will give clues for the direction of intervention for the treatment personnel.

Development of the "curious" attitude is best done through practice. Because transference and countertransference issues are revealed to the client over time, ongoing consultation with other trusted professionals provides the necessary input to counterbalance blindspots created by the clinician's own history. In this, health care professionals can be more clear about their own boundaries and can offer clients more thorough, objective, and compassionate understanding of their idiosyncratic boundary issues.

SUMMARY

This paper has reviewed four areas for the professional to develop in order to complete excellent assessments. They are (1) familiarity with boundary inadequacies as an issue for recovering clients; (2) personal preparation in the form of self-examination;

(3) respect for individual differences; and (4) practice, in consultation with respected and knowledgeable professionals.

Developing this expertise will enable the clinician to accomplish the three-fold goal of boundary inadequacy assessment: (1) to develop a unique understanding of the clients and their histories with boundaries; (2) to pinpoint areas of boundary inadequacies whose treatment is integral to successful recovery from chemically dependent family systems; and (3) to aid clients in self-understanding which encompasses themes of independence, dependence, interdependence, power, caring, and respect for individual differences.

When these goals are reached in a successful assessment, the clients can begin to view themselves with understanding rather than shame. From this basis of self-referenced information shared with a professional, the clients can begin or continue the process of healthy recovery from patterns of ambiguous, overly rigid, or invasive boundary inadequacies. This appears to be essential for successful recovery from chemically dependent systems.

REFERENCES

Beckman, L.J. (1984). Treatment needs of women alcoholics. *Alcoholism Treatment Quarterly*, 1(2), 101-114.
Coleman, E. & Colgan, P. (1986). Boundary inadequacy in drug dependent families. *Journal of Psychoactive Drugs*, 18(1), 21-30.
Coleman, E. & Schaefer, S. (1986). Boundaries of sex and intimacy between client and counselor. *Journal of Counseling and Development*, 64, 341-344.
Colgan, P. (1987). Treatment of dependency disorders in men: Toward a balance of identity and intimacy. *Journal of Chemical Dependency Treatment*
Filstead, W.J. (1984). Gender differences in the onset and course of alcoholism and substance abuse. *Alcoholism Treatment Quarterly*, 1(1), 125-132.
Finkelhor, D. (1981). Common features of family abuse. Paper presented at Research Conference on Family Violence, Durham, NH.
Johnson, C., & Flach, A. (1985). Family characteristics of 105 patients with bulimia. *American Journal of Psychiatry*, 142(11).
Kaufman, G. (1974). The meaning of shame: Toward a self-affirming identity. *Journal of Counseling Psychology*, 21(6), 568-574.
Maddock, J. (1975). Sexual health and health care. *Postgraduate Medicine*, 58(1).
Mason, M., & Fossum, M. (1986). *Facing shame*. New York: W. W. Norton.
Montagu, A. (1971). *Touching: The human significance of skin*. New York: Harper & Row.
Neilsen, L.A. (1984). Sexual abuse and chemical dependency: Assessing the risk for women alcoholics and adult children. *Focus on Family*, Nov-Dec.

Schaefer, S., & Evans, S. (1984). The incest continuum: A conceptual framework for assessing incestuous dynamics and behaviors in families. Paper at International Institute on the Prevention and Treatment of Alcoholism. Athens, Greece.

Smalley, S. (1982). *Co-dependency: An introduction*. New Brighton, MN: SBS Publications.

Solomon, R.L. (1980). The opponent-process theory of acquired motivation. *American Psychologist*, 35(8), 691-712.

Woititz, J.G. (1983). *Adult children of alcoholics*. Hollywood, FL: Health Communications, Inc.

Wolin, S.J., Bennett, L.A., & Noonan, D.L. (1979). Family rituals and the recurrence of alcoholism over generations. *American Journal of Psychiatry*, 136(4B), 589-593.

Women, Sexuality and the Process of Recovery

Susan Schaefer, MA
Sue Evans, MA

SUMMARY. This paper discusses the importance of addressing sexuality issues in the treatment of chemically dependent women. It summarizes the research which has correlated chemical dependency in women to such areas as: sexual dissatisfaction/dysfunction, sex role conflicts, intimacy and interpersonal relationships, sexual orientation issues and sexual abuse/incest. Four primary factors impacting the relationship between women's sexuality and recovery will be explored including: social influences, physical correlates, psychological components and spiritual aspects. This paper draws on existing research, the authors' clinical experience, and information provided to the authors by the self-reports of 100 chemically dependent women who were extensively surveyed. This paper should be viewed as both an invitation to others for further research into these relationships, as well as a challenge to alcoholism and mental health professionals to incorporate more aspects of sexuality work into the individual treatment plans and overall treatment programs for their recovering women clients.

Kate, a 33-year-old computer programmer, recently admitted herself for chemical dependency treatment. Having used alcohol and pills daily for the past two years, Kate decided she needed help with her addiction. While in treatment, Kate reported to her

---

Susan Schaefer is a licensed psychologist and certified chemical dependency practitioner in private practice in Minneapolis, MN. Sue Evans is a certified chemical dependency practitioner and an AASECT-certified sex educator and is also in private practice in Minneapolis.

Requests for reprints can be sent to Susan Schaefer, MA, at 2400 Blaisdell Avenue South, Minneapolis, MN 55404.

© 1987 by The Haworth Press, Inc. All rights reserved.

counselor that she often felt numb during sex, experiencing few sensations at all. She stated that she found herself oftentimes feeling panicky before and during sexual activities with her partner—terrified by sexual intimacy. Due to this terror, Kate regularly got "high" before engaging in sex. Kate admitted to her counselor that she was generally dissatisfied with her sexual relationships and acknowledges that she often bartered herself sexually for companionship and affection. Kate had rarely experienced sex without the use of mood-altering chemicals and now had great concern for her recovery.

Kate's story is similar to that of countless other women seeking treatment for alcoholism and drug dependency. Increasingly as treatment counselors begin asking clients direct questions related to sexuality, they are discovering the need to devote more time clinically to addressing these issues in treatment and aftercare programs. It has been found that sexuality is important to address in chemical dependency treatment because it is such an integral part of a chemically dependent woman's recovery (Sterne, Schaefer and Evans, 1983). Many women who have not dealt with their sexuality in prior treatments report returning to chemical use in order to protect themselves from painful feelings surrounding their sexuality in areas such as sexual dissatisfaction/dysfunction, sex role conflicts, intimacy and interpersonal relationships, sexual orientation issues, and sexual abuse/incest (Evans and Schaefer, 1980).

SEXUAL DISSATISFACTION/DYSFUNCTION

The sexual concerns of chemically dependent women have been acknowledged for several decades, although early studies are scarce and reflect biases in sex role stereotyping. A common example of this may be seen in studies where women are referred to as promiscuous while men with similar histories of sexual activity are said to be engaged in frequent extramarital affairs (as noted by Wilsnack, 1982). A number of studies discuss "promiscuity" as an integral aspect of the alcoholic woman's psychological makeup—without defining the term (Hart, 1930; Curran, 1937; Karpman, 1948; Levine, 1955 and Meyerson, 1959). The later work of Schuckit, (1972) and Browne-Mayers, Seelye and

Sillman (1976) served to debunk this myth as each found that sexual acting out behavior applied to only 5% of alcoholic females. Similarly, in a survey of 100 chemically dependent women, Evans, Schaefer and Sterne (in preparation) found the majority of their sample of 100 women in recovery did not fit the promiscuity myth. The median number of sexual partners per year reported by the women for a five year period prior to their seeking treatment was 1.8.

While historically alcoholic women were often thought to be sexually suspect, loose or in fact prostitutes, recent research points to inhibited sexual desire and responsiveness as a far more frequent problem (Kinsey, 1966 and 1968: Blane, 1968; Schuckit, 1972 and Browne-Meyers et al., 1976). For some women sexual dysphoria and dysfunction may be linked to the long-term side effects from the chemicals themselves. For others the chemicals may have been used to cope with or mask sexual problems that preceded the onset of chemical abuse. Kinsey (1966) reported that 72% of his sample of female alcoholics stated that "frigidity" preceded and contributed to their drinking problem while 79% of Covington's (1982) sample of chemically dependent women stated they experienced sexual problems before alcohol use became a concern for them.

Clearly there appears to be a strong relationship between chemical use and sexuality. The exact nature of that relationship, however, is a complex one. Athanasiou (1970) found that 68% of the females in his study (opposed to 45% of the males) reported that alcohol heightened their sexual enjoyment. While the aphrodisiac qualities of alcohol have been touted since time immemorial, Shakespeare's Macduff[1] was perhaps the first to most accurately describe the limitations of this aphrodisiac when he described it provoking the desire, but taking away from the performance. Indeed Macduff's anecdotal observations are borne out in the research of Wilson and Lawson (1967 and 1978) who found that women reported experiencing higher levels of sexual arousal (subjective response) with increased blood alcohol levels. However, their physiological responses as measured by a vaginal photoplethysmograph (objective response) indicated lower arousal levels. Malatesta, Pollack, Crotty and Peacock (1982) later corroborated this finding as well.

SEX ROLE CONFLICTS

A number of researchers have found that chemically dependent women experience sex role confusion as a factor in their alcoholism. Kinsey (1966) reported that alcoholic women suffer an inadequate adjustment to adult female sex roles. Parker (1972) found among the alcoholic women studied that despite their sex role preferences being more traditionally masculine in terms of occupation, attitudes and interests, when drinking, they expressed more traditional female behaviors. Wilsnack (1973) found the opposite to be true as she discovered that some alcoholic women accept the traditional feminine role as gratifying on a conscious level but in fact are quite traditionally masculine (assertive, independent) on an unconscious level and experience this as an inability to fulfill society's expectations. She proposed that some women drink to ease this conflict. In a follow-up study of non-alcoholic women, Wilsnack (1974) found that these women tended to drink to feel more feminine, sexy, warm and expressive. Still later, Wilsnack (1976) suggested that it doesn't really matter in which direction the conflict occurs (feminine/conscious, masculine/unconscious) rather it is the sex role conflict per se which is important as a stress factor in women's alcoholism.

INTIMACY AND INTERPERSONAL RELATIONSHIPS

In their sample of chemically dependent women, Schaefer, Evans and Sterne (1985)[2] found that typically the interpersonal context within which sexual activity had occurred was not satisfactory. It could be characterized as: (1) lacking in mutuality, (2) failing to meet intimacy needs, and marked by (3) the woman's lack of trust for her partner, (4) her inability to communicate what pleased her sexually, and (5) her feeling of powerlessness to control whether or not she engaged in sex. This is not surprising since the alcoholic woman's conditioning both as to women's sexual role within the larger culture and to her often rigidly defined sex role within an alcoholic family system affects the adult sexual role that she adopts. In an age of seeming liberalization of sexual norms and changing roles for women, it is important to note that many of the women seen in treatment were educated to believe that sex is shameful, dirty, sinful and to be feared; that men enjoy it and women do not, and that it is a way women can please others.

Lack of mutuality is expressed in these women's recognition that they have been exploited, and are objects for their partners' pleasure rather than valued as a person in their own right:

> I thought men were out for their own satisfaction and didn't care if they hurt me. I didn't think I had any needs — my part was to please and satisfy men. I felt they only wanted me for sex, not interested in me personally. When they got bored with me, they went away. I felt having sex was the only way a man should be interested in me.[3]

Where the lines between affection, intimacy and sexuality are blurred, women may seek to obtain the former two by engaging in the latter. Yet they come to realize that something is missing:

> It was too sexual . . .no trying to know one another.[3]
>
> . . . the few encounters I've had were shallow, over quick, left me feeling more lonely than before.[3]

Lack of trust, itself a factor in the inability to establish intimacy, is often based on a history of exploitation. More than half the women studied had a history of childhood sexual abuse, primarily intrafamilial. Some felt very detached during sexual encounters and went through the motions with little emotional involvement or sexual feelings. Lack of trust was also explicitly connected to an inability to "let go" sexually and experience sexual satisfaction.

In their orientation toward pleasing and caretaking, many alcoholic women showed little awareness of what is sexually pleasing to them personally. Even when they do have some awareness, the social conditioning of their passivity makes it difficult to communicate needs — sexual or otherwise.

For a variety of reasons, alcoholic women may feel powerless to control the circumstances under which they have sexual relations. Some of these include: a loss of control and psychological vulnerability experienced while intoxicated, sex role definitions which do not support self-assertion, and patterns of victim behavior ingrained from histories inundated with emotional, physical, or sexual violations. All of these combine to create the perception among many recovering women that they do not have personal rights or decision-making power.

SEXUAL ORIENTATION

Early psychoanalytic thinking held the hypothesis that alcoholism was often associated with unresolved issues of homosexuality. This belief was held during a period in which homosexuality was generally believed to be pathological. During the early 1970s, as attempts were being made to challenge the premise that homosexuality was pathological and remove it from the diagnostic and statistical manuals which categorized nervous and mental disorders, Saghir (1973) undertook a study to address the mental health of lesbian women in comparison to heterosexual women. In assessing these two groups on a number of variables related to mental health, Saghir found that the groups differed on only two variables: lesbian women were seven times more likely to drink to excess than their heterosexual counterparts and four times as likely to have been suicidal. These researchers were not able to find differences between the groups on other measures of psychological adjustment.

Others have since corroborated these higher rates of addiction among homosexual men and women. Swanson, Loomis, Lukesh, Cronin and Smith (1972) reported four times the rates of addiction to alcohol, barbiturates and amphetamines in a group of lesbian women as compared to a control group. Fifield (1975) reported 30% of the lesbian/gay population she surveyed in Los Angeles admitted to chemical use, a finding later replicated in a Midwestern survey (Lohrenz, 1978).

SEXUAL ABUSE/INCEST

During the early to mid 1970s treatment centers were beginning to report that 40-50% of their female clients had experienced incest in their backgrounds (Evans and Schaefer, 1980). These early reports, based on clinical observations and informal surveys, were soon substantiated by research. In a study of 188 female patients being treated for alcoholism, Benward and Denson-Gerber (1975) found that 44% had experienced incest in their past. Similarly, in a comparison study by Schaefer, Evans and Sterne (1985), 39% of the sample of chemically dependent women (N = 100) cited prior histories of incest while 24% of a control group reported the same.

FACTORS IMPACTING THE RELATIONSHIP BETWEEN WOMEN'S SEXUALITY AND RECOVERY

The relationship between women's sexuality and recovery is a composite of many factors. This section addresses four primary areas, including social influences, physical correlates, psychological components and spiritual aspects which affect this relationship.

Social Influences

In order to understand the relationship between chemical dependency and sexuality for women, it is necessary to look to the larger social structure which impacts this relationship. Particularly in providing therapy to women attempting to heal from issues related to sexuality and addiction, it is important to place each woman's personal history within the context of her socialization. In doing so, one may come to understand what appears to be one woman's own brand of "craziness" may simply be a reasonable response to an unreasonable environment.

In addition to society, the family serves as another primary educator regarding the teaching of appropriate chemical use, tools for dealing with emotions, communication patterns, degree of intimacy allowed, sexual rules and regulations, respect for its members' boundaries and ultimately, what is socially acceptable behavior for little girls and boys. The socialization process begins immediately at birth exerting a strong influence. For example, it is still common practice for female infants to receive pink stocking caps and blankets and boys to receive blue within minutes after birth to maintain body temperatures. The innocent pink or blue cap becomes a symbol for the differential expectations parents impart, as progenitors of society at large. In understanding the relationship between women's chemical use and sexuality then, it is helpful to consider some of the unique societal demands and sex role expectations placed on her in this culture.

This society worships a cult of beauty and youth. In women's attempts to live up to this image of perfection, many experience poor self-concepts along with an inordinate amount of body shame. This is often compounded by a sense of failure and worthlessness especially if she feels unable to attract men. There is evidence that both men and women suffer under pressures to perform when confined by rigid adherence to narrow sex role standards. These pressures produce anxiety, low self-esteem, and serve to restrict adaptability and self-expression (Bem, 1974).

Traditionally, masculinity has been closely associated with being unemotional, aggressive, dominant, decisive, and competent. In sexual matters, men have been expected to be the initiator, in a constant and uncontrollable state of arousal, and focused on genitalia and goals. On the other hand, traditional femininity has been closely associated with emotionality, passivity, submission, indecisiveness, and learned helplessness. In sexual matters, women have been trained to be process-oriented reactors with few of their own sexual needs, placators, "keepers of the virtue"; while at the same time taught to be responsible for their partner's sexual satisfaction with little attention or validity afforded to their own sexual fulfillment and trained to compete with and mistrust other women.

> I'm not real sure of what "sexuality" even means. I feel I have so much to learn — some things I have never thought or talked about. I believed my role was to be a wife and satisfy a man, keeping him so he wouldn't stray. My duty was to "submit myself unto my husband."[3]

Research has indicated that women more than men feel their alcoholism is precipitated by a major life crisis which, not so coincidentally, often revolves around their roles as women (Lisansky, 1957; Curlee, 1969). Crises such as death of a spouse, marital difficulties, post partum depression, menopause and children leaving the home ("Empty Nest Syndrome") are often noted as precursors to women's heavy drinking periods.

Additionally, self-destructive behavior patterns arise out of the conflicting double standard for what it is to be a woman. Particularly ambiguous is the role of women's sexual identity, with the virgin/whore dichotomy a common message for women to receive. This dichotomy, while experienced by all women to some extent, is certainly felt even more by chemically dependent women who often are stigmatized as promiscuous. It is common to see in treatment groups some women expressing great shame for having had too many sexual experiences while others in the same group express equal amounts of shame for having had too little (Evans and Schaefer, 1980).

> I thought that now that I've finally done it (sex), I don't have the right to say no anymore. Under this assumption I became active with many partners and lost some self-esteem and power.[3]

> I don't feel sexual. I do it mainly because "I should." Not satisfactory. No fun. I'd give myself a C−.[3]

Sex Role Ambiguity

Wilsnack (1976) found that the potential female alcoholic has chronic doubts about her adequacy as a woman and undergoes conflicts due to a lack of congruity between her conscious and unconscious values and traits regarding male/female roles.

Just as some women drink to get in touch with their femininity, others may drink to get in touch with their masculine (traditionally defined) qualities such as strength, assertiveness and personal power. In a society where women are relatively powerless, one of the few areas where they can feel power is through their sexuality. Women are taught that sexuality, in fact, is their tool for power. They learn to both use and withhold sex to get what they need—using sex as barter for touch, protection, security, affection, companionship or love. They are taught sex is something given to, done to or for them, reinforcing their powerlessness.

The rigid adherence to restrictive sex roles when taken to its extreme may well account for the high incidence of sexual abuse/incest among chemically dependent women. Old practices of male ownership of women and children continue to get enacted through such over-subscriptions to sex roles and other manifestations of "gynephobia" which run rampant in society and are expressed daily to women in the form of sexual harassment on the job, being propositioned on the street, being pinched, rubbed up against, raped through coercive, marital or stranger rape or sexually violated by a family member.

> I only see sex as a situation of control and dominance (one of) victim/victimizer. Having an orgasm means losing control, it doesn't feel safe.[3]

Unfortunately all too often societal sex role demands and expectations predispose women to self-destructive behavior patterns which frequently, directly or indirectly, involve chemical use/abuse. While some women begin abusing chemicals at an early age and continue on with chronic patterns of chemical abuse which eventually result in dependency, other womens' relationships with chemicals may be more indirect. For this second group it is common to see periods of serious chemical abuse interspersed with periods of abstinence while being involved with an alcoholic partner, only to resume unhealthy patterns of chemical abuse after the breakup of their relationship. In both cases women experience a continuous relationship with the chemical even though they may not be personally ingesting it.

PHYSICAL CORRELATES

Often the physical effects of the drugs themselves preclude the possibility of chemically dependent women living up to the myth of promiscuity which continues to shroud their image. Much to the contrary, the growing body of research on women and addiction points to the obverse, namely, the effect of alcohol and other drugs is often quite disruptive to female sexual response and functioning. Current reports indicate that chemical usage in mod-

arousal capacity, (2) orgastic dysfunction, (3) lubrication impairment, and (4) loss of libido (Dowsling, 1980). (See Wilsnack [1982] for a review of related studies.) Alcohol, marijuana, cocaine, amphetamines, narcotics and hallucinogens have all been implicated, as well as a host of prescription medications including oral contraceptives, antihistamines and even the alcohol antagonist, Antabuse (see Table I.)

Explanations of the possible physiological mechanisms through which chemicals affect sexual functioning have been offered by Whitfield, Redmond and Quinn (1979). These include: (1) the general depressant effects of alcohol and other drugs which numb sensation leading to arousal, (2) disruption of the delicate hormone balance caused by liver damage which interferes with arousal and orgastic ability, (3) sensory neuropathy which blocks sexual arousal, (4) organic brain damage which can result in a loss of sex drive, and (5) secondary medical problems known to interfere with sexual functioning such as hypertension, diabetes, depression and vaginitis.

In addition to the specific effects alcohol and other drugs have on women's sexual functioning, when expanded to include broader aspects of female sexuality (obstetric-gynecological concerns) far greater effects are incurred from the use of both prescription and non-prescription drugs. Previously little information about these effects has been available to the lay public or among human service professionals working with women in recovery. This information, important to the practice of human service professionals of many disciplines (social work, chemical dependency, psychology, etc.) has also not been readily available in traditional training programs. As a result, few clinicians are equipped to deal with cases in their clinical practice which reflect these concerns.

Table I shows the variety of effects which can occur with the use of different categories of prescription drugs. Not all drugs within each category listed produce listed effects. To determine which specific medications produce these effects, consult a physician, Physician's Desk Reference, or refer to DeMoya, DeMoya, Lewis and Lewis (1982); Story (1974).

In addition to the effects of prescription medication, research-

Table I

Prescription Drug Effects on Female Sexuality

Potential Effects on Female Sexuality	Categories of Drugs Prescription
1. Breast Enlargement	Anti-hypertensive Medication with Diuretic, Anti-depressants
2. False Pregnancy Testing	Anti-psychotics, Appetite Suppressants
3. Uterine Bleeding	Anti-anxiety Medication
4. Enlargement of Clitoris	Anabolic Steroids
5. Galactorhea - Excessive Breast Secretion	Anti-psychotic and Anti-anxiety Medication
6. Irregular Menses	Anti-psychotics, Appetite Suppressants, Anti-hypertensive Medication and Diuretics
7. Mastalgia - Painful Breasts	Anti-anxiety Medication
8. Amenorhea - Cessation of Menstrual Period	Anti-anxiety Medication
9. Lactation - Production of Milk from Breast	Anti-psychotics, Anti-hypertensive Medication
10. Alteration of Secondary Sex Characteristics - Masculinization with voice deepening and hair growth	Anti-hypertensive Medication with Diuretic, Anabolic Steroids

ers have linked alcohol abuse to reproductive and gynecological problems including:

1. Abnormally high menstrual irregularities and dysmenorrhea linked to chemical abuse (Podolsky, 1963; Belfer, 1971; Benjafield and Rutter, 1972; Wall, 1937; Beckman, 1979; Wilsnack, 1982).
2. Higher rates of drinking among premenstrual women (Beckman, 1979).
3. Fluctuating rates of blood alcohol levels and corresponding rates of intoxification with different phases of the menstrual cycle. The premenstrual phase producing the highest peak of blood alcohol with same quantity of alcohol (Jones and Jones, 1976).
4. Reduced rate of alcohol metabolism found for women on oral contraceptives (Jones and Jones, 1976; Sutker, 1982).
5. Significantly more gynecological surgery (other than hysterectomy) for subgroups of heavier drinking women (Wilsnack, 1982). Since it is not known to what degree drinking increases the need for gynecological surgery compared to what extent women use alcohol to cope with gynecological problems, Wilsnack notes that further research is needed to address the nature of this correlation.
6. Harmful effects on the developing fetus (Fetal Alcohol Syndrome): chemical usage by pregnant women has been shown to affect the birthweight, intelligence, nervous system and physical development of the unborn child (Jones, Smith, Ulleland and Streissguth, 1973; U.S. Department of Health, Education and Welfare, 1977; Clarren and Smith, 1978; Little, 1982).

Additionally, infertility, repeated miscarriage, stillbirths, premature births and difficult labors have also been correlated with women's chemical abuse (Kinsey, 1968; Benjafield and Rutter, 1972; Wilsnack, 1973).

Although much of the research on women's sexual/reproductive functioning is fraught with methodological problems (small sample size, lack of control groups and difficulty separating cause and effect) these studies seem to suggest a correlation between alcohol cravings and hormonal status. However, there is also research which disputes this (Lisansky, 1957; Driscoll and Barr, 1972; McNamee, Grant, Ratcliffe, Ratcliffe and Oliver, 1979).

Regardless of the conflictual data, the authors have long noted chemically that women in recovery are at the highest risk for relapse during the premenstrual phase of their cycles. This, obviously, can be due to a number of reasons: hormonal changes, psychological stress, physical discomfort. What is described as premenstrual syndrome (PMS) in the literature no doubt plays a major role as a risk factor in relapse.

Premenstrual syndrome has been described to be caused by cyclical hormonal imbalances (Light, 1984). The estrogen-progesterone imbalances alter carbohydrate metabolism which can in turn produce symptoms such as tension, fatigue, headaches, dysphoria, cravings for sugar, more food or alcohol. For a chemically dependent woman, PMS may simply be an exacerbation of a condition (malfunctioning carbohydrate metabolizing system) she experiences throughout the month.

The symptoms of PMS are similar to those of low blood sugar (hypoglycemia). Currently, the treatment of PMS incorporates the treatment for hypoglycemia as well.

As the blood sugar drops, the symptoms can be physical (shakiness, headaches), intellectual (loss of memory, disruption in concentration), or emotional (irritability, depression). The symptoms result from the brain not getting enough fuel to function as it becomes glucose starved. As the blood sugar drops, cravings for alcohol/sugar are the body's misguided attempt at restabilization.

Morton (1953) found that for women in general, the lowest point in their blood sugar is at the premenstrual phase of their cycles (low or flat glucose tolerance curves). For alcoholic women especially, the low blood sugar symptoms may be exacerbated by PMS, causing her to crave alcohol/sugar which can result in a relapse.

One study which addresses both sexual functioning and biochemical stabilization was conducted by Benjafield and Rutter (1972). In a seven year investigation of the biochemical and genetic factors in 44 male and 21 female long-termed abstinent alcoholics, the following was reported in relation to the female sample: longstanding menstrual irregularities, infertility, anorgasmia, oophorectomy and hysterectomy. Among the biochemical factors noted were: flat blood glucose curves, raised androgen and lowered estrogen levels and enzyme defects in carbohydrate metabolism.

It is possible that teaching women to chart their menstrual cycles and to be particularly careful about their diet and vitamin regime during the premenstrual phase of their cycle can be helpful in preventing relapse.

Beyond the specific relationship between low blood sugar and PMS which has implications for women in recovery is the more general relationship between alcoholism itself and hypoglycemia which has been described by a number of professionals in the field. Tintera (1966) wrote: "In the alcoholic, whether predisposed, active or recovered, the prevailing factor is hypoglycemia." Cheraskin (1974) followed with: "Alcoholics report during low blood sugar periods they crave alcohol, coffee, nicotine and sweets." Similarly Lieber (1976) reported: "Low blood sugar or hypoglycemia is known to be a complication of acute alcoholism but is often overlooked." Moreover, alcoholics experience disproportionately high rates of hypoglycemia: 95% (Meiers, 1973), 96% versus 14% for a control group (Poulos, 1976).

In general, the treatment programs that address nutritional restabilization for men and women have higher rates of recovery as reported by Fredericks, 1976; Mindell, 1979; and Covington, 1985.

The current treatment for hypoglycemia and PMS consists of a diet, exercise and vitamin program. Refraining from sugar, white flour and caffeine is the first step. Secondly, eating six small snacks throughout the day rather than three large meals is helpful. Thirdly, eating complex carbohydrates rather than refined, processed foods is important. Finally, adequate amounts of protein is required.

Exercise is also an important component of the restabilization process. Aerobic exercise—minimally 20 minutes in duration 3 times a week unless medically restricted—helps stabilize the blood sugar (Bailey, 1977).

These preliminary studies and our clinical observations point to the necessity of addressing physical stabilization as part of the recovery process in therapy. Clinicians need to be asking their clients about, drawing correlations to, gathering more information on and making appropriate referrals for the restabilization of biochemical imbalances.

This should be dealt with during each phase of treatment and recovery. The authors offer the following guidelines:

Assessment Phase: Assist client in noting links between her chemical use, menstrual cycle, and acting out behaviors.

Treatment: Require a referral to a physician for a thorough physical exam complete with a six hour glucose tolerance test. Work with each client to establish (either directly or through referral) a healthy dietary, nutritional and exercise program—one based on the individual needs and medical constraints of each client.

Aftercare: Encourage the client to keep a journal noting the relationship between periods of adherence to the diet/exercise program she has worked out versus periods she has gone off this program.

SHAME

Most chemically dependent women come from chemically dependent families themselves where they have grown up in a shame-based family system (Coleman, 1983; Nielsen, 1984). They start out with an identity that is characterized by a core feeling of unworthiness, low self-esteem and a demeaned self-concept. While feelings of having nothing to offer and of never quite measuring up are experienced generally they are increased in relation to the addictive process.

Chemical dependency is often referred to as a "feelings disease." It is characterized by a general repression of emotions by finely tuned defense mechanisms. Out of their need to protect themselves from exposure and vulnerability, chemically dependent women tend to build thick walls around themselves and master a variety of defenses in an effort to feel safe and avoid the risk of exposing their true selves to others (which they perceive as deserving ridicule and mockery). This fear of exposure which produces shame, is paralleled and intensified with respect to sexuality and interferes with the potential for intimacy.

> I am currently feeling asexual and at times an aversion to sex. I do not want sexual relations at all—with anyone. Those times during which I have felt interest or sexual arousal I subverted or ignored. Now I feel as though I have stuffed those feelings so often that I am incapable of deep physical attachment.[3]

Through the use of chemicals one's emotional complexion can be repressed, altered or intensified. It is, however, unlikely that persons can selectively pick and choose which feelings they wish to block or gain access to. It can be argued that in attempting to numb out one side of the emotional continuum, such as anxiety, pain or grief aspects of the other end of the continuum get suppressed as well: the potential for delight, arousal, elation.

Similarly, if chemicals are used to get in touch with those feelings which are normally repressed (i.e., the woman who is only able to orgasm while drunk) those same chemicals may well access a host of negative feelings such as abandonment, paranoia, disappointment or fear. Just as no chemical exerts a specific desired action on the body exclusively, so it is that no chemical is capable of calling forth any one desired feeling state and many women who attempt to utilize alcohol as a survival tool to manage their feelings soon find it blocks their self-growth.

Once sober, with chemicals no longer available to serve as crutches, the chemically dependent woman may find her defenses returning full force. This is why traditional, "heavy confrontative, male-model" type of chemical dependency treatment is not appropriate for most women. These defenses were developed for a reason and to crack them open with "hot seat" tactics without regard to what the defenses might be protecting is not conducive to healing. Women need to be supported and encouraged out of their defenses. When pushed into a corner, shame-based women know easily how to become compliant or defiant— neither of which facilitates work on the underlying issues: issues which may include unresolved feelings related to past sexual abuse experiences, sexual dysfunction or what is the most common intimacy concern expressed by women in recovery—fear of sex sober.

> I feel very sad about my sexuality. I've been taught that it's something I can't have, I'm afraid of it. I fear no gratification and I fear that I don't perform well. I have been told by men that I have a low sex drive. I have compensated in the past by faking it.[3]

GUILT

A second psychological factor affecting the relationship between women's sexuality and recovery is guilt. Most often this is experienced in conjunction with a changing value system or behaviors experienced while intoxicated which violated old codes of morality. As chemical use progresses and the chemically dependent woman feels more and more powerless, many areas of her life become unmanageable, including those related to value systems. Sexual practices accompanying her chemical use (using sex to get drugs/alcohol, poor partner choices, or even just being physically more vulnerable to sexual abuse while drunk) often does not fit her sober value system. This conflict produces guilt and anxiety. With anxiety attached to her sexual performance she may find herself unable to engage in satisfying sexual relationships which over time begin to erode her sexual self-concept. "I feel inadequate because I am not in control of my orgasms."[3]

Many women turn to more chemicals to deal with this problem but find when chemicals are used to medicate feelings they often interfere with more successful conflict resolution. It is easy at this point for self-destructive patterns to escalate.

DEPRESSION

One of the significant differences between chemically dependent men and women is the corresponding rates of depression. Women in recovery experience more than 5 times the rates of primary depression as their alcoholic male counterparts (Cadoret and Winokur, 1974). Primary depression may be defined as depression which occurs prior to the onset of heavy chemical abuse and may include organic (biochemical) or functional (stress related) depressions. Certainly some of the functional depression experienced by women in recovery beyond that caused by the immediate stressors in their lives may well be linked more generally to their role as "second class citizens" in society. The impact of depression on a women's sexuality typically involves a loss of interest, motivation and drive; with many depressed women defining themselves as "sexless" or "asexual."

Another common element experienced by women is a sense of learned helplessness. As usage continues, a greater sense of unmanageability, powerlessness and frustration all combine with the consequences of her use to create a sense of helplessness which nurtures a growing depression and decreases the likelihood of healthy self-expression — sexual or otherwise.

This learned helplessness also impacts women by promoting the "victim role" which often gets manifested in destructive relationships. (For more discussion of the victim role see "Incest and the Chemically Dependent Woman: Treatment Implications" in this volume [Evans and Schaefer, 1987].)

GRIEF

A major portion of a chemically dependent woman's recovery often centers around grieving. Common types of grief issues include: loss of self-image, loss of missed opportunities, loss of an ideal family and loss of their chemical. With respect to sexuality, there are also many losses to be grieved: loss of innocence, loss of romantic myths, loss of virginity, loss of sober values, loss of relationships along with the losses which come out of grieving past sexual abuse. Additionally, many women grieve their differences (by their interpretation, deviations from the perceived sexual norm).

Grieving often continues years into a woman's recovery. There are four major aspects of this grieving process: (1) recognizing and admitting the losses (cognitive), (2) affirming the pain of the losses to self and others (emotional), (3) freeing self from the bondage of deprivation by filling the voids and restoring oneself (psychological), and (4) defining new possibilities for growth and self-actualization (spiritual).

The losses of childhood, including normal sexual development, are quite clear to many newly recovered women. It is apparent to many clinicians that many recovering women experience an arrested psychosexual development at approximately 12-14 years of age or the age they began drinking, and need to "go back" and reclaim the part of themselves that stopped growing at the onset of their chemical usage. It is a difficult but often exciting process for women to begin to reclaim their sexuality.

> It's exhilarating—this feeling of newness. I've always been using before this point in time so all of my sexual development and experience was influenced by my alcoholism. Here I am, sober, 22, and I'm 15 and just discovering myself at the same time. What nervousness! What joy![3]

SPIRITUAL ASPECTS

One of the main tasks of recovery is to search out harmony and integration of all the basic needs of the self. An integral part of this process for women is to reclaim the spiritual aspects of themselves. Alcoholics Anonymous is a helpful tool in this regard for many women in recovery but additional methods are needed due to the highly personal and complex nature of each woman's search for her spirituality. An important part of this process is to look for the "blockers" (Many of which traditionally have been defined as involving sexuality) and "accessors" of this search for spirituality whether through orthodox religious or non-traditional efforts.

Spirituality, like women's sexuality, has been historically associated with male guides, be they spiritual leaders or lovers. Women have been taught that they are not capable of directly accessing either their spirituality or sexuality which reinforces their powerlessness and male dependency. Many orthodox religious beliefs involve strong strictures regarding appropriate sexual behavior. Most often sexuality and spirituality are posed as dichotomous and often competing human needs. In order to obtain spiritual enlightenment women have been instructed they must either abstain from sexual expression or follow rigid codes of conduct, i.e., sex only within marriage, sex only for procreation, sex appropriate only with men, sex as duty or moral obligation.

With these rules many women come to feel they must suppress their sexuality in order to become spiritual while others, unfortunately, feel they must suppress their spirituality in order to become sexual. "Sometimes I feel God is angry at me for being sexual."[3]

A great amount of shame and guilt is often associated with these beliefs in order to maintain the sanctions and social order. Women in particular have assumed an inordinate amount of shame for simply being women. For centuries women's menses have been regarded as unclean and sapping her and those around her of spiritual power. Many myths and rituals and religious practices have originated out of this fear of women's power. To this day, few religions allow women to become spiritual leaders.

The roles women are given from religious history seem to offer few choices within which to express spirituality and sexuality. The Virgin Mary and prostitute Mary Magdalene offer almost archetypal images of the dichotomous roles offered to women (virgin/whore). While these strong culturally inspired images serve to stereotype and restrict sexual roles for women in general, alcoholic women carry an even heavier burden in being unfairly typecast and sexually stigmatized as loose, impetuous and amoral in their sexual behavior.

For many recovering women, their behavior while using chemicals served to (especially in the area of sexuality where the latitude of sanctioned expression is very limited) cut themselves off from the traditional sources of their spirituality, i.e., organized religion. As their disease progressed and chemical use became out of control, new behaviors were experienced which no longer fit their sober value system. With this ethical deterioration the old sense of morality and spirituality often gave out with little to replace it but self-hatred, doubt and shame.

An additional element in this process to consider is the effect of drugs not only on behavior but the introspective process itself, which is intimately tied to one's spirituality. Drugs, especially the hallucinogens, are often used in attempts to artificially elicit spiritual enlightenment and promote spiritual growth. Unfortunately, in most cases the use of chemicals only served to distance users from their spiritual source or offer capricious, non-sustained insight which typically wears off with the "high." Over time many women have experienced a sense of disillusionment in this form of spiritual questing.

By the time many chemically dependent women enter treatment, then, they are out of touch with their God and without a belief, not only in a "higher power," but themselves as well. The beginning period of recovery is often one of disenchantment, isolation and alienation from religious orthodoxy, one's spiritual self and any higher power – a general state of existential and spiritual despair.

An important part of recovery, then, for many women is owning and reclaiming their spirituality, either by coming to some reconciliation with their traditional religious beliefs or discovering their own. Through their spiritual recovery women often come to realize they, too, have a heritage they can be proud of: one that comes from a long line of mothers, healers, birthers, herbalists and growers – in touch with the cyclical nature of themselves and the world. For many women recovery means learning to distinguish their *own* inner voice – not the voice of reason, not the voice of their parents or a shaming culture, not the voice of "their victim" (that says over and over to abuse themselves). Their inner voice is, instead, the "voice of their spirit." It involves the power to intuit. It is the voice which teaches them to quietly and firmly push away their "extraneous voices" and to trust their "own voice." Out of this healing process often comes the need to create new spiritual rituals.

With respect to sexuality, the challenge that awaits women in recovery is to integrate their visions of sexual health with their newfound spirituality. In doing so they might well come to question whether or not spirituality and sexuality originate from the same energy source, a part of themselves that is pure and clean and whole. In viewing themselves in such a light sexuality could be viewed as a generalized life force rather than a localized sensation, one where sexuality and spirituality are intricately interwoven in their day-to-day lives rather than a contradiction of terms (Evans and Schaefer, 1980).

ADDENDUM I

Basic Assumptions of a Women's Sexuality Group in a Treatment Setting

1. Women-only group.
2. It is important to structure the group format with lecture/information, group exercises and individual assignments to help the women counter the "no talk rule." It is also helpful to find a balance between education and feelings work as both are crucial. The exercises and assignments can act as a catalyst for this.
3. The goal of the group is (sexual) empowerment for women. Encourage self-direction, helping women to take their sexual power back and to trust themselves. Let each woman determine the depth of her sharing (with only *gentle* confrontation when needed) and encourage bonding with other group members.
4. Address holistic recovery:
   — emotional healing
   — intellectual learning
   — physical restabilization
   — spiritual wholeness
5. Provide clear and unambiguous rules in the group to clarify boundaries, offer structure and increase trust:
   a. Confidentiality.
   b. Minimum time commitment required.
   c. No violence or threats allowed (to self or others).
   d. Two-week notice for closure.
   e. No sexual contact between group members.
   f. No chemical use allowed.
   g. Each woman is responsible for her own therapy:
      i. Asking for time.
      ii. Being timekeeper for someone else.
      iii. Giving honest feedback/confrontation.
      iv. Being responsible for fulfilling or negotiating assignments.
I. Socialization
   A. Women's sexuality as a feminist issue.

1. Many sexual barriers stem from culturally learned attitudes and stereotypes.
   a. Sex roles and their limitations.
   b. Traditional masculinity/femininity training.
   c. Double messages:
      —virgin/whore
      —frigid/promiscuous
      —victim/victimizer
2. Sex as a power tool/barter system for women.
3. Help women put their own experience into societal context (not their particular sickness).
   B. Help women realize they now have choices/options beyond their social training.
II. Reclaiming Sexual Power
   A. Women are trained to give away sexual power.
      1. Faking orgasm.
      2. Lying with their bodies.
      3. Caretaking partners.
      4. Being afraid of being "whorish."
      5. Being passive—"Sex is something done to them."
   B. Taking back sexual power is hard work.
      1. Fantasies/erotic dreams.
      2. Assertiveness training/communication skills.
      3. Self-nurturing/self-focusing.
      4. Boundary work.
      5. Body work:
         a. masturbation/sensate/focus.
         b. massage.
      6. Define sexuality/sensuality/intimacy and give themselves one of each.
      7. Spiritual connections.
III. Genitalia
   A. Body parts and functions.
      1. Many women lack knowledge of genital structure and/or don't know what pleases them.
      2. Exploration and investment to gain knowledge and familiarity (and pleasure):
         a. vulva picture.
         b. masturbation.

B. Body Shame
C. Gynecological Considerations
1. Birth control methods.
2. Abortion.
3. Menstruation and menopause.
4. Medical concerns.
5. Sexually transmitted diseases.
IV. Childhood Sexuality
A. First sexual memories.
B. What our parents taught us about sex/intimacy/touch.
C. Masturbation/sex play.
D. Touch needs.
E. Any shame/guilt?
F. Any abuse or boundary violations?
V. Adolescent Sexuality.
A. Developing bodies.
B. Menstruation.
1. How did you learn about it?
2. Do you have any feelings about it?
C. Self-Image.
D. Role Models.
E. Relationships.
1. Fears and fantasies.
2. Peer pressure.
3. Parental/family response.
F. Virgin/Whore Conflict.
VI. Boundary Ambiguity/Clarification.
A. Boundary Development (in childhood).
B. Boundary Violations.
1. Emotional.
2. Physical.
3. Sexual.
C. Effects of Boundary Violations.
D. Reclaiming Boundaries.
VII. Sexual Abuse.
A. Continuum of abuse.
1. Every woman has been abused in some way.
a. Put it within the social context of dominance and submission.

         b. Abuse is often connected to her use.
     B. Resulting fear of intimacy.
     C. Healing oneself from the abuse.
VIII. Effects of Chemical Dependency on Female Sexuality.
     A. Physiological Effects.
         1. Disrupt delicate hormone balance.
         2. Anesthetize sensations.
     B. Repression of emotions — Chemical dependency is feelings disease.
     C. Shame based family system.
     D. Common sexual concerns of chemically dependent women.
         1. Inability to orgasm.
         2. Loss of interest in sex.
         3. Lessened inhibitions while using.
         4. Low self-esteem.
         5. Prostituting self for drugs.
         6. Being vulnerable to sexual abuse while using.
IX. Sexual Identity Issues.
     A. Rates of chemical abuse among gays/lesbians.
         1. Recovering women often question their sexual attractions.
     B. Homophobia/biphobia.
         1. Ingrained since birth — values conflict.
         2. Guilt and shame of living lifestyle with no social or religious sanctions.
         3. Stress of integrating public/private life.
         4. Self-hatred.
         5. Possible family alienation.
     C. The Continuum of Affectional Preference.
         1. Kinsey Scale.
         2. Fluidity of lifestyle choices.
         3. Normalize feelings.
X. Integrating Spirituality and Sexuality
     A. Organized religions teach that they are mutually exclusive.
     B. Alcoholic behaviors cut one off from spiritual connections.
     C. Need to become aware of own spiritual connection.

1. Sexuality and spirituality arise out of same energy source.
2. Can heal ourselves – develop our own power, and attend to own inner voice.
3. Power outside of ourselves to draw upon.
   a. Women's heritage of birthers, nurturers, healers, mothers.
   b. Cycles of nature and ourselves.
   c. Women nurturing women.
   d. Higher power in whatever form we find it.
D. New Models of Sexual Health.

This model can also be utilized as an aftercare group or a general sexual therapy group. Structure group discussion every 4-6 weeks by drawing from the main topic areas of the outline. The rest of the time encourage each woman to talk about her own issues. This allows for structure and content of the group process while allowing each woman to be responsible for her own therapy.

NOTES

1. *Macbeth*.
2. Written in collaboration with Muriel Sterne, appeared in: *Sexuality Issues Affecting Women in Recovery*. Minnesota Chemical Dependency Association Newsletter, Vol. 3, No. 4, pp. 3-4, April 1985.
3. This quote and all others are actual. The authors wish to acknowledge the recovering women of their study whose quotes appear throughout this paper. They also extended their gratitude to Chrysalis Center for Women where the study was conducted and to co-researcher Muriel Sterne.

REFERENCES

Abel, E. L. (Ed.). *Fetal Alcohol Syndrome* (Vol. 2: Human studies; Vol. 3: Animal studies). Boca Raton, FL: CRC Press, 1982.
Amir, M. "Alcohol and Forcible Rape." *British Journal of Addictions*, Vol. 62: 219-232, 1967.
Athanasiou, R., P. Shaver and C. Tavris. "Sex: A Psychology Today Report." *Psychology Today*, Vol. 4: 39-52, 1970.
Bailey, C. *Fit or Fat*. Boston: Houghton Mifflin Co., 1977.

Beckman, L. J. "Reported Effects of Alcohol on the Sexual Feelings and Behavior of Women Alcoholics and Non-alcoholics." *Journal of Studies on Alcoholism*, Vol. 40 (3): 272-282, 1979.
Belfer, M. L., R. I. Shader, M. Caroll and J. S. Harmatz. "Alcoholism in Women." *Archives of General Psychiatry*, Vol. 25: 540-544, 1971.
Bem, S. L. "The Measurement of Psychological Androgyny." *Journal of Consulting Clinical Psychology*, Vol. 42: 155-162, 1974.
Benjafield, J. G. and L. F. Rutter. "Diagnostic Tests in Alcoholism." *British Journal of Addictions*, Vol. 67: 231-234, 1972.
Benward, J. and J. Densen-Gerber. "Incest as a Causative Factor in Antisocial Behavior: An Exploratory Study." *Contemporary Drug Problems*, Vol. 4: 323-340, 1975.
Blane, H. T. *The Personality of the Alcoholic: Guises of Dependency*. New York: Harper and Row, 1968.
Browne-Mayers, A. N., E. E. Seelye and L. Sillman. "Psychosocial Study of Hospitalized Middle Class Alcoholic Women." *Annals of the New York Academy of Sciences*, Vol. 273: 593-604, 1976.
Cadoret, R. and G. Winokur. "Depression in Alcoholism." *Annals of the New York Academy of Sciences*, Vol. 233: 34-40, 1974.
Cavallin, H. "Incestuous Fathers: A Clinical Report." American Journal of Psychiatry, Vol. 134: 1132-1138, 1966.
Cheraskin, E., N. M. Ringsdorf and A. Brecher. *Psychodietetics*. New York: Bantam, 1974.
Clarren, S. K. and D. W. Smith. "The Fetal Alcohol Syndrome." *New England Journal of Medicine*, Vol. 298: 1063-1067, 1978.
Coleman, E. "Sexuality and the Family: Effects of Chemical Dependence and Codependence on Individual Family Members" in P. Golding (Ed.), *Alcoholism: Analysis of a World-Wide Problem*. Lancaster, England, MTP Press Limited, 1983.
Colgan, P. and E. Coleman. "Chemical Dependency Among Patients Treated for Sexual Concerns." Unpublished manuscript, 1979.
Covington, S. S. "Nutritional Factors Affecting Alcoholism." *Anabolism*, p. 4, Winter, 1985.
Covington, S. S. "Sex and Violence — The Unmentionable in Alcoholism Treatment." Paper presented at the National Alcoholism Forum of the National Council on Alcoholism. Washington, D.C., 1982.
Curlee, J. "Alcoholism and the 'Empty-Nest.'" *Bulletin of the Menninger Clinic*, Vol. 33: 165-171, 1969.
Curran, F. G. "Personality Studies in Alcoholic Women." *Journal of Nervous and Mental Diseases*, Vol. 86: 645-667, 1937.
DeMoya, A., D. DeMoya, M. Lewis and H. Lewis. *Sex and Health: A Practical Guide to Sexual Medicine*. Stein and Day Publishing Co., 1982.
Dowsling, J. L. "Women: Alcoholism and Sexuality." Paper presented at the National Council on Alcoholism, Seattle, WA: May, 1980.
Driscoll, G. Z. and H. L. Barr. "A Comparative Study of Drug Dependence and Alcoholic Women" in *Selected Papers of the 23rd Annual Meeting of Alcohol and Drug Problems of North America*, pp. 9-20, 1972.
Evans, S. and S. Schaefer. "Why Women's Sexuality Is Important to Address in Chemical Dependency Treatment." *Grassroots: Treatment and Rehabilitation*, pp. 37-39, 1980.
Fifield, L. "On My Way to Nowhere: Alienated, Isolated and Drunk." Los Angeles Gay Community Service Center Research Project, 1975.
Fredericks, C. *Psychonutrition*. New York: Grosset and Dunlap, 1976.

Hart, H. H. "Personality Factors in Alcoholism." *Archives of Neurology and Psychiatry*, Vol. 24: 116-134, 1930.

Henn, F. A., M. Herjanic and R. H. Vanderpearl. "Forensic Psychiatry: Profiles of Two Types of Sex Offenders." *American Journal of Psychiatry*, Vol. 133 (6): 694-696, 1976.

Jones, B. M. and M. K. Jones. "Women and Alcohol: Intoxification, Metabolism and Their Menstrual Cycle." In M. Greenblatt and M. A. Schuckit (Eds.) *Alcoholism Problems in Women and Children*. New York: Grune and Stratton, 1976.

Jones, K. L., D. W. Smith, C. N. Ulleland and A. P. Streissguth. "Pattern of Malformation In Offspring of Chronic Alcoholic Mothers." *Lancet*, Vol. 1: 1267-1271, 1973.

Karpman, B. *The Alcoholic Woman*. Washington, D.C.: Linacre Press, 1948.

Kinsey, B. A. *The Female Alcoholic: A Social Psychological Study*. Springfield, IL: Charles C. Thomas, 1966.

Kinsey, B. A. "Psychological Factors in Alcoholic Women from a State Hospital Sample." *American Journal of Psychiatry*, Vol. 124: 1463-1466, 1968.

Levine, J. "The Sexual Adjustment of Alcoholics: A Clinical Study of a Selected Sample." *Quarterly Journal of the Study of Alcohol*, Vol. 16: 675-680, 1955.

Lieber, C. S. "The Metabolism of Alcohol." *Scientific American*, Vol. 234 (3): March, 1976.

Light, M. H. "Premenstrual Tension." *Homeostasis Quarterly*, March, 1984.

Lisansky, E. S. "Alcoholism in Women: Social and Psychological Concomitants: I. Social History Data." *Quarterly Journal of the Study of Alcohol*, Vol. 18: 588-623, 1957.

Little, R. E., J. M. Graham, H. H. Samson. "Fetal Alcohol Effects in Humans and Animals." *Advances in Alcohol and Substance Abuse*, Vol. 1 (3/4): 103-125, 1982.

Lohrenz, L. J., J. C. Connelly and K. E. Spare. "Alcohol Problems in Several Midwestern Homosexual Communities." *Journal of Studies on Alcohol*, Vol. 39: 1959-1963, 1978.

Malatesta, V. J., R. H. Pollack, I. D. Crotty and I. J. Peacock. "Acute Alcohol Intoxification and Female Orgasmic Response." *Journal of Sex Research*, Vol. 18 (1): 1-17, 1982.

McNamee, B., J. Grant, J. Ratcliffe, W. Ratcliffe and L. Oliver. "Lack of Effect of Alcohol on Pituitary-Gonadal Hormones in Women." *British Journal of Addiction*, Vol. 74: 316-317, 1979.

Meiers, R. C. "Relative Hypoglycemia in Schizophrenia," in Hankins, O. and L. Pauling (Eds.), *Orthomolecular Psychology*. San Francisco: W. H. Freeman, 1973.

Mindell, E. *Vitamin Bible*. New York: Warner Books, 1979.

Morton, J. A. "A Clinical Study of Premenstrual Tension." *American Journal of Obstetrics and Gynecology*, Vol. 65: 1182, 1953.

Myerson, D. J. "Chemical Observations on a Group of Alcoholic Prisoners." *Quarterly Journal of the Study of Alcohol*, Vol. 20: 555-572, 1959.

Nielsen, L. A. "Sexual Abuse and Chemical Dependency: Assessing the Risks for Women Alcoholics and Adult Children." *Focus on Family*, p. 6, Nov.-Dec., 1984.

Parker, F. B. "Sex Role Adjustment in Women Alcoholics." *Quarterly Journal in the Study of Alcohol*, Vol. 33: 647-657, 1972.

Podolsky, E. "The Woman Alcoholic and Premenstrual Tension." *The Journal of American Medical Women's Association*, Vol. 18: 816-818, 1963.

Poulos, J., D. Stafford and K. Carron. *Alcoholism, Stress and Hypoglycemia*. New York: Sterling Publications, 1976.

Rada, R. T. "Alcoholism and the Child Molester." *Annals of the New York Academy of Sciences*, Vol. 273: 492-496, 1976.
Saghir, M. T. and E. Robins. *Male and Female Homosexuality: A Comprehensive Investigation*. Baltimore: Williams and Wilkins, 1973.
Schaefer, S., S. Evans and M. Sterne. "Sexual Victimization Patterns of Recovering Chemically Dependent Women." *Proceedings of the International Institute on the Prevention and Treatment of Alcoholism*. Calgary, Alberta, Canada: August, 1985.
Schuckit, M. "Sexual Disturbance In the Woman Alcoholic." *Medical Aspects of Human Sexuality*, Vol. 6: 44-62, 1972.
Sterne, M., S. Schaefer and S. Evans. "Women's Sexuality and Alcoholism," in P. Golding (Ed.), *Alcoholism: Analysis of a World-Wide Problem*. Lancaster, England, MTP Press Limited, 1983.
Story, Norman L. "Sexual Dysfunction Resulting from Drug Side Effects." *The Journal of Sex Research*, Vol. 10 (2), 132-149, May, 1974.
Sutker, P. E. "Acute Alcohol Intoxication: Mood Changes and Gender." Paper presented at the 13th Annual Medical-Scientific Conference of the National Alcoholism Forum, Washington, D.C., April, 1982.
Swanson, D. W., S. P. Loomis, R. Lukesh, R. Cronin and J. A. Smith. "Clinical Features of the Female Homosexual Patient." *The Journal of Nervous and Mental Diseases*, Vol. 155 (2): 119-124, 1972.
Tardiff, G. "La cuminalite de violence." M.A. Thesis, University of Montreal, 1966.
Tintera, J. W. "Stabilizing Homeostasis in Recovered Alcoholics through Endocrine Therapy: Evaluation of the Hypoglycemia Factor." *Journal of American Geriatrics Society*, Vol. 14 (2): 1966.
Tintera, J. W. and H. A. Lovell. "Endocrine Treatment of Alcoholism." *Geriatrics*, Vol. 4 (5): September, 1949.
U.S. Department of Health, Education and Welfare, Press release, June 1, 1977.
Wall, J. H. "A Study of Alcoholism in Women." *American Journal of Psychiatry*, Vol. 93: 943-952, 1937.
Wilsnack, S. C. "Alcohol, Sexuality and Reproductive Dysfunction in Women" in E. L. Abel (Ed.), *Fetal Alcohol Syndrome, Vol. II*. CRC Press, 1982.
Wilsnack, S. C. "Sex Role Identity in Female Alcoholics." *The Journal of Abnormal Psychology*, Vol. 82: 253-261, 1973.
Wilsnack, S. C. "The Effects of Social Drinking on Women's Fantasy." *Journal of Personality*, 42: 43-61, 1974.
Wilsnack, S. C. "The Impact of Sex Roles on Women's Alcohol Use and Abuse" in Greenblatt, M. and M. A. Schuckit (Eds.) *Alcoholism Problems in Women and Children*. New York: Grune and Stratton, 1976.
Wilsnack, S. C. and L. J. Beckman (Eds.). *Alcohol Problems in Women*. New York: Guilford Press, 1982.
Wilson, G. T. and D. M. Lawson. "The Effects of Alcohol and Sexual Arousal in Women." *Journal of Abnormal Psychology*, Vol. 85: 489-497, 1967.
Wilson, G. T. and D. M. Lawson. "Expectancies, Alcohol and Sexual Arousal in Women." *Journal of Abnormal Psychology*, Vol. 87: 358-367, 1978.
Whitfield, C. L., A. C. Redmond and S. J. Quinn. "Alcohol Use, Alcoholism and Sexual Functioning." Unpublished manuscript, University of Maryland School of Medicine, 1979.

Sexual Orientation Concerns Among Chemically Dependent Individuals

Susan Schaefer, MA
Sue Evans, MA
Eli Coleman, PhD

SUMMARY. The rates of alcoholism among the gay/lesbian and bisexual population has been estimated to be three times that of the general public. The socio-political influences that produce higher rates of alcoholism are reviewed. Specific issues in the treatment of chemically dependent men and women are defined and specific suggestions to address sexual orientation issues in treatment and the recovery process are made.

The National Council on Alcoholism and the National Institute of Alcohol Abuse and Alcoholism currently estimate that ten percent of the general population in the United States is alcoholic. Among the gay/lesbian/and homosexual population, the rates of alcoholism have been estimated to be three times that of the general public (Fifield, 1975; Lohrenz, Connelly & Spare, 1978).

Since the early 1900s, a perceived correlation between alcohol abuse and homosexuality has been described in the psychological and psychiatric literature (Small & Leech, 1977). During the first half of the century a number of psychoanalytically-based theories

---

Susan Schaefer is a licensed psychologist and a certified chemical dependency practitioner in private practice in Minneapolis, MN. Sue Evans is a certified chemical dependency practitioner and an AASECT-certified sex educator and is also in private practice in Minneapolis. Dr. Coleman is Associate Director and Associate Professor at the Program in Human Sexuality.

Requests for reprints can be sent to Susan Schaefer, MA, at 2400 Blaisdell Avenue South, Minneapolis, MN 55404.

© 1987 by The Haworth Press, Inc. All rights reserved.

have been put forward to explain this connection. These theories posited the view that:

1. Compulsive drinking served as a defense against sexual inadequacies (male) and penis-envy (father).
2. Latent homosexuality could more easily become manifested under the disinhibiting influence of alcohol.
3. Alcoholic relationships were often based on oral fixations that most typically involved same-sex relationships.
4. Homosexuality resulted from a phobic reaction to being heterosexual and could be mollified through the use of alcohol.

These early theories were based on clinical observations, and once subjected to the rigors of experimental analysis, little evidence emerged to support them (Prout, Strongin & White, 1950; Botwinick & Machover, 1951; Gibbins & Walters, 1960; McCord & McCord, 1960.) Other serious shortcomings of the psychoanalytic theories were identified that eventually led to their demise:

1. Since many theories spoke to the relationship between latent homosexuality and alcoholism, it could be inferred that alcoholism and homosexuality were mutually exclusive, with manifest homosexuality serving as a deterrent to alcoholism. This inference appears to contradict the very basis upon which the theories were derived.
2. Many theories addressed the psychosexual development of males and were couched in male terminology. The psychoanalytic theories did not speak to the relationship between female homosexuality except through possible extrapolation.

With the onset of gay liberation in the late 1960s, research on homosexuality took a new direction, one that challenged the belief that homosexuality could be considered a psychiatric illness. The earliest systematic studies designed to evaluate the psychological health of homosexuals versus that of heterosexuals came out of what may be referred to as the modern era of research on homosexuality (see Hooker, 1957). Originally, the studies of the early 1970s set out to establish a comparison between homosexuality and heterosexuality on a variety of psychological dimensions, including affective disorders, anxiety-phobic neuroses, alcoholism, drug abuse, hysteria, psychopathic behavior, obsessive compulsiveness, paranoia, and schizophrenia. Results of these studies indicated no statistically significant differences between the two groups, except for a significantly greater incidence of alcoholism and drug abuse among the homosexual comparison groups (see Gonsiorek, 1977, for a review of this literature).

Saghir, Robins, Walbran, and Gentry (1973), and Swanson, Loomis, Lukesh, Cronin, and Smith (1972) compared a group of lesbian women to a control group of heterosexual women with respect to a number of psychological variables. Overall, no statistically significant differences were observed in the psychological adjustment between the two groups except that lesbians showed a greater prevalence of alcoholism and usage of nonprescription medications. Additionally, lesbians exhibited a higher incidence of depression and suicide attempts that were shown to be directly related to their use of alcohol and drugs.

Similarly, in a study of the differences in rates of psychopathology between gay and heterosexual men, Saghir, Robins, Walbran, and Gentry (1973) found a higher proportion of gay men reported using marijuana, amphetamines, hallucinogens, amyl nitrite, barbiturates, opiates, and alcohol. In studying over 2,000 gay men from several countries, Weinberg and Williams (1974) also concluded there were no significant differences in the psychological problems of gay men compared with heterosexual men except with respect to drinking. Twenty-nine percent of the gay men in this study reported alcohol abuse.

Whereas these early studies were aimed at comparing gays and lesbians to heterosexuals on a variety of psychological variables, more recent studies have been aimed specifically at studying rates of alcoholism in the gay community.

Fifield (1975), using a number of procedures including self-reports, bartender questionnaires, private interviews and the Blood Alcohol Content Index (a legal device for measuring intoxification), concluded that fully one-third of the total gay population of Los Angeles County abused alcohol on a regular basis.

More recently, Lohrenz and his associates (1978), in a study of alcoholism among gay men of four midwestern states, found that 29 percent were alcoholic.

Finally, in the years since the Fifield study, reports from a number of gay counseling clinics in Pittsburgh, Philadelphia and Los Angeles, as well as surveys of professionals who treat gay alcoholics, have corroborated the finding that one out of every three gays and lesbians experience alcohol abuse or alcoholism (Ziebold and Weathers, 1975). Nardi (1982), however, notes that there have been serious methodological flaws in the studies described above and that no systematic, rigorous epidemiological survey of alcoholic or of drinking patterns exist. There is some evidence that this population may be at higher risk. (For further discussion of the history and review of the literature see Nardi, 1982.)

The research of Beckman (1979), Sterne, Schaefer, and Evans (1984) and Covington (1982) has included information on the proportion of chemically dependent women who are bisexual. The results ranged from 3 percent (Beckman) to 20 percent (Covington). As noted by Sterne, Schaefer, and Evans (1983), the proportion of women who identify themselves as being heterosexual, bisexual or lesbian is often quite different from a purely behavioral analysis of their sexual behavior. The resulting disparity between one's stated identity and actual sexual behavior may produce intrapsychic conflicts that chemicals later serve to medicate, and this phenomenon can have important implications for treatment.

As mentioned earlier, the onset of the gay liberation movement resulted in a political and social movement that ultimately had a profound effect on the psychiatric and psychological community. The result was in a change of focus in the research on homosexuality: the focus moved from studying intrapsychic variables related to homosexuality (Illness Model) to exploring extrapsychic variables that influence gay/lesbians and affect their adjustment in society (Stress Model). This model emphasized socio-political aspects of being gay or lesbian that effect adaptation, adjustment, and health. This change of focus ultimately led to the 1973 decision that homosexuality *per se*, be removed from the Diagnostic and Statistical Manual for Mental Disorders by the American Psychiatric Association.

SOCIO-POLITICAL INFLUENCES PRODUCING HIGHER RATES OF ALCOHOL ABUSE

There are many socio-political influences that produce higher rates of alcohol abuse among gays and many socio-political aspects to being gay, lesbian, or bisexual in a heterosexual society. Three general ways in which society influences rates of alcohol abuse or alcoholism will be described here, and then each will be discussed in terms of how it operates in the gay/lesbian/bisexual community and contributes to the disproportionately higher rates of alcohol abuse and alcoholism. Finally, the psychological correlates of each of these factors will be addressed.

Three major ways in which a culture or society influences rates of alcoholism are (Bales, 1946; Snyder, 1959):

1. The degree to which the culture operates to bring about acute needs for adjustment or inner tensions in its members.
2. The attitude toward drinking that the culture adopts.
3. The degree to which the culture provides suitable substitute means of satisfaction.

In reference to the first of these factors, it is reasonable to assume that living with the daily pressures of a lifestyle that is not socially accepted creates tremendous tensions and adjustment difficulties; thus gay, lesbian, and bisexual individuals carry a stigma that leads to alcohol abuse or alcoholism. Bisexual and lesbian women, of course, carry an additional stigma: that of being a woman, which results in an even greater compounding of guilt and shame. A homophobic and biphobic culture serves to discount, humiliate, invalidate, and alienate its gay, lesbian and bisexual members, which (apart from its own destructiveness) becomes internalized into self-hatred. Departure from heterosexual roles ingrained from infancy produces serious value conflicts. Finally, the stress associated with coming to grips with one's sexual orientation—along with the constant search to integrate one's private and public life with a minimum of punitive repercussions—creates overwhelming pressures, which individuals often medicate with chemicals. As Ziebold (1979, p. 39) said, "Homosexual individuals who have been forced to develop rigid defenses against social reaction to their sexual and affectional orientation may unknowingly let these same reflexes reinforce a budding dependency on alcohol." In another vein, society is responsible for the subliminal and sometimes often overt traumatization of gay/lesbian/and bisexual individuals. It has been noted by Coleman (1987a) that chemical dependency and family intimacy dysfunction are inextricably bound. Societal intolerance and covert or overt abuse of alcohol can be equated with family abuse or trauma. Therefore, Coleman's (1986b) hypothesized model of the development of compulsive behaviors, including chemical abuse, can apply (see Figure 1.) Note that either family abuse, or trauma, or societal or cultural intolerance or abuse can set the stage for the development of compulsive behaviors (e.g., chemical abuse). When an individual experiences both family abuse or trauma and societal or cultural intolerance, these individuals are at even higher risk for developing compulsive behavior patterns (see also Quadland, 1985).

In regard to the second factor, bars serve as the traditional meeting places for gay/lesbian and bisexual persons. This is both a cultural promotion and a subcultural acceptance of drinking as the main means of socialization.

The bar scene lends itself to the use of anxiety-releasing and disinhibiting effects of alcohol or other drugs. Reliance on or abuse of alcohol and other drugs can circumvent the experiencing of feelings and the resolution of conflict which is necessary for identity integration (see Coleman 1981/82). Alcohol or other

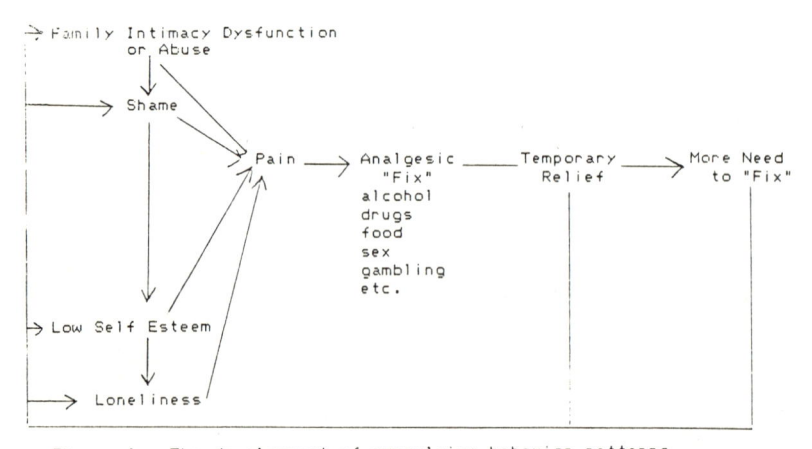

Figure 1. The development of compulsive behavior patterns.

drugs can provide a temporary feeling of well-being, intimacy, or identity integration, which is dependent upon a particular situation (e.g., in a bar under the influence of alcohol or other drugs). For many, it is easy for them to feel comfortable with their sexuality under the influence of alcohol and in the relative safety of a homosexually identified bar; but in the light of day, interacting with a predominately heterosexual society, the feelings can be quite different (see also Monegon and Ziebold, 1982; and Ziebold, 1978).

The compulsive use of the "bar scene" can serve as a transitional phase or can become a stopping place where an individual remains fixated at an identity development stage that usually precludes identity integration.

With respect to the third factor—the degree to which the culture provides suitable means of satisfaction—few alternatives to bars have existed for gay, lesbian, and bisexual individuals seeking ways in which to socialize with others without fear of reprisal. Fortunately, this sociological situation is changing in most urban areas, with the growth of social, political, and religious organizations. These organizations are providing other opportunities for socializing.

In summary, there are three ways in which a given society influences rates of alcoholism; (1) the degree to which the culture operates to bring about acute needs for adjustment in its members; (2) the attitudes toward drinking fostered by the culture; and (3) the degree to which alternative forms of tension-reducing activities are available; each operates more powerfully on the lesbian and gay community members and contributing to higher rates of alcoholism.

SPECIAL TREATMENT CONSIDERATIONS

Chemical dependency counselors and other human service professionals need to be sensitive to even the most subtle expressions of biphobia and homophobia. For many of us, our training has been laced with homophobic theories and practices. As mentioned earlier, it was not until 1973 that the American Psychiatric Association removed homosexuality from its diagnostic and statistical manual for mental disorders. It returned ego-dystonic homosexuality in DSM III, leaving some vestiges of the illness notion of homosexuality.

Most psychotherapists have been introduced to counseling theories that, at the very least, discount same-sex relationships (Garfinkle and Morin, 1978). The language and basic assumptions of the chemical dependency field especially do not speak to alternative lifestyles. For example, chemical dependency counselors often assume "he" is the alcoholic and "she" is the codependent. The family systems approach used by many therapists is often confined to the intact, stereotypical family (which, in reality, according to the Bureau of Labor Statistics accounts for only 17 percent of Americans). Seldom is the family systems approach broadened in such a way so as to include, and thereby validate, the relationships and new-found families of the gay/lesbian/bisexual client. Seldom are the same-sex "spouses"/partners/lovers given the same invitation to become involved in treatment as are the husbands and wives and other family members upon whom the family systems approach was derived (Schoener, 1976). Additionally, as counselors have become sensitized/educated to gay rights/liberation, they have oftentimes ignored and shamed bisexuals who face an inordinate pressure to conform to either end of the Kinsey continuum.

As chemical dependency counselors gain new attitudes toward bisexual and homosexual clients, new messages will conflict with the old ones we all carry as members of a society that does not award religious, social, or legal sanctions to its non-heterosexual members. This conflict typically creates a certain amount of cognitive dissonance in counselors. There are several ways in which we can resolve the dissonance we experience as we attempt to integrate the old and new messages. We can:

1. Deny our feelings of discomfort.
2. Choose not to relate to that part of the client (ignore sexual orientation issues).
3. Change our relationship with the client (transfer him or her to another therapist).
4. Attempt to change the client (get him or her to be more heterosexual).

5. Begin to change our attitudes and beliefs about bisexual and homosexual individuals.

The manner in which we resolve our attitudes will directly affect the quality of services we are able to provide.

Biphobia and homophobia are found not only in the culture but are also deeply ingrained and internalized in the same-sex person as well. As individuals come to grips with sexual identity issues, they often face a tremendous amount of fear, guilt, shame and alienation. Due to the extreme psychological vulnerability resulting from these feelings, it is a high risk time for chemical abuse. As the client increasingly becomes more aware of the difference between himself or herself and the mainstream of society, he or she may escape this pain through an even greater involvement with alcohol and drugs.

In treatment, then, it is absolutely essential that clients be able to not only deal with the harmful consequences of drug use but also with the feelings they have about their identity, sexuality, and lifestyle, all elements that are intimately related to the use of alcohol and other drugs. If they are unable to deal with these issues in the context of treatment, the chances for a quality sobriety are minimal.

It has been noted by Colcher (1982) that some homosexual clients come into treatment stating emphatically that they do not have any problem regarding their homosexuality, but after testing and trusting their counselors, they will begin to talk openly about their feelings.

Gay/lesbian and bisexual individuals need to be encouraged to talk about their fears and pain in a trusting and safe therapeutic environment. They can best be encouraged to begin this critical portion of their therapy through the gentle support of a caring, understanding and validating therapist.

Encouraging clients to feel good about their emerging sexual orientation identity and lifestyle is a process that needs to be individualized to best fit each client's unique history, circumstances, expectations and goals. Each person has his or her own internal timing that allows for the necessary steps toward self-acceptance. To attempt to accelerate this time frame is often counter-therapeutic. The client's sense of knowing when to move to the next step should be respected. The process of "coming out" can be used to illustrate this point. The political aspects of coming out are complex (DeCecco, 1980). Even for persons who are not politically active, coming out has inevitable indirect political repercussions. Counselors working with gay/lesbian and bisexual individuals need to have a basic understanding of these issues in order to provide meaningful services. Encouraging some people to come out as soon as possible may not be advisable therapeutically. For others, coming out can be a liberating step in fostering a sense of pride and self-acceptance.

It is important for counselors to remember that the fear individuals face in coming out to family, friends or work colleagues is often based on reality. Each time an individual comes out, he or she faces the risk of being misunderstood, discriminated against, ostracized, or physically harmed. The client needs to weigh each new situation and arrive at a decision he or she can feel comfortable with. The counselor can be helpful in sorting through each situation as well as processing what is best for each person at a given time, ultimately respecting the choice he or she makes.

SEXUAL ORIENTATION ISSUES IN RECOVERY

Inherent in the perceptions of heterosexual, bisexual and homosexual persons are certain stereotypes that, when applied to individuals within each group may seem accurate but do not readily apply to the group as a whole. Many of the stereotypes operate to produce fears or phobias. These fears are best dealt with in a therapeutic sexuality group, where they can be discussed and where barriers between individuals can be broken down. Heterosexuals speak of their fear of being sexually approached by non-heterosexuals in the group. Gay men and lesbians often talk about an unwillingness to trust heterosexuals for fear of being exploited. Both groups may share a fear of getting close to the bisexuals, who are often seen as "shallow opportunists." Each phobic response may be grounded in a real (past) experience. Within a sexuality group, these issues emerge and need to be addressed before trust will develop to the extent that any real therapeutic work can take place.

The therapist's role at this time should be to assist clients in taking back their power and working to help them move from a posture that is passive-victim-restrictive to one which is active-creative-constructive (see Smith, 1979). Some may be encouraged, depending on their readiness and willingness to become involved with political and social activism, to change from internalizing pain to converting their intense feelings into an energy that has an external, positive focus (e.g., volunteering to work at a battered women's shelter), organizing a "Take Back the Night" march, or working with a gay/lesbian/bisexual rights group.

Once sobriety has become stabilized, clients often raise sexual orientation issues. Often persons going through treatment begin to feel intimacy with others of the same or opposite sex for the first time in their lives. Sometimes this newfound feeling of warmth and closeness is confusing; the differences between affection, intimacy, and sexuality become blurred.

For those beginning to explore sexual attractions to others of their own sex—as well as for those who feel they don't quite fit into any sexual category—the ability to see sexual orientation as a continuum rather than a category can be helpful. This premise is based on the information gathered by Kinsey and his associates (1948, 1953).

Kinsey originally questioned subjects not only about their overt sexual behavior but also about their psychic reactions. The important point that Kinsey and his associates made, and one about which counselors need to be continually reminded, is that sexual orientation is complex and can not be divided into the simple dichotomous categories of homosexual and heterosexual. Kinsey and his associates found that sexual orientation must be viewed on a continuum. They developed a 7-point scale (in which 0 represented exclusive heterosexuality and 6 represented exclusive homosexuality) to better understand sexual orientation. (See Figure 2.)

In terms of the scale, Kinsey et al. (1948) reported that a third of the persons studied fell within the middle 1-5 range.

The Kinsey Scale has proved to be a helpful framework within which to help clients begin to explore their sexual orientations. As part of this process, sexuality, like many other aspects of a

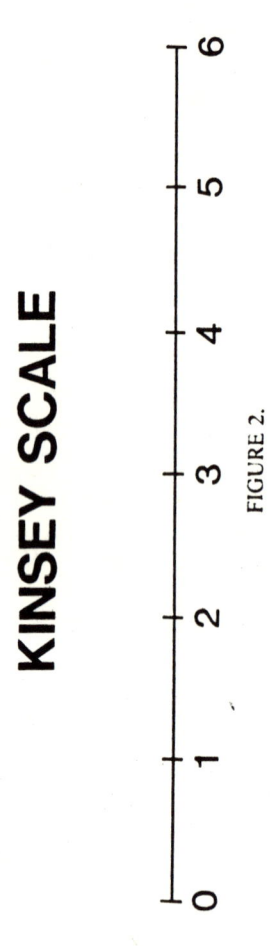

KINSEY SCALE

0 — 1 — 2 — 3 — 4 — 5 — 6

FIGURE 2.

person, may involve changing definitions over the years. Viewing affectional preference as a continuum rather than a category allows room for this flux.

Although the continuum concept is helpful, it should be noted that there are both advantages and disadvantages to adopting a specific sexual orientation identity. On the one hand, it can produce feelings of pride, joy, and strength as well as an identity which can bring support and a sense of solidarity and community. The drawbacks of adopting a category are the unwritten rules and regulations that inhibit feelings and limit choices about who one is attracted to, where one can get support, and what constitutes a politically correct way to behave (DeCecco, 1980).

Trying to fit within the confines of a given category is particularly difficult for bisexual individuals, who often are the most cautious and confused about their sexual feelings, since they have been raised with the belief they must choose between being straight or gay/lesbian. "Bisexual women face many of the same pressures as lesbian women, but unlike lesbians, bisexuals have no discernible subculture, no developed political base, and less in common with each other sexually than either heterosexual or lesbian women" (Orlando, 1978).

Like homosexual men and women, bisexual individuals come from diverse backgrounds and have great differences in personality, developmental experiences, and relationship patterns. For some, their bisexuality is transitional—a bridge between heterosexuality and homosexuality. For others, it is sequential-relationships with men during a given period of their lives and with women during another period. For still others, their bisexuality is historical; they live a predominantly heterosexual lifestyle but have had some past experiences in same-sex relationships (see Klein, 1978). Some bisexual individuals however, have concurrent relationships with both men and women. Out of these concerns about over-simplification, Coleman (1986) has developed a clinical tool that can be used by clinicians to better assess or help a client assess his or her sexual orientation (see Table 1). This assessment device uses nine dimensions of sexual identity. The first dimension is a descriptor of life style or current relationship status.

Secondly, the client is asked to identify their current sexual orientation. Thirdly, they are asked to identify what they would like their sexual orientation to be in the future. Fourthly, they are asked to give a global assessment of comfort or self acceptance of their current sexual orientation identity.

Beyond these dimensions, this model measures four more dimensions, including the four components of sexual identity (physical, gender, sex-role, and sexual orientation in terms of the

TABLE 1

ASSESSMENT OF SEXUAL ORIENTATION

© Eli Coleman, Ph.D.

1986

Name or Code Number: Age: Date:

What is your current relationship status:

○ Single, no sexual partners

○ Single, one committed partner Duration

○ Single, multiple partners

○ Coupled, living together (Committed to an exclusive sexual relationship)

○ Coupled, living together (Relationship permits other partners under certain circumstances)

○ Coupled, living apart (Committed to an exclusive sexual relationship)

○ Coupled, living apart, (Relationship permits other sexual partners under certain circumstances)

○ Other

In terms of my sexual orientation, I identify myself as . . .	In the future, I would like to identify myself as . . .
○ Exclusively homosexual	○ Exclusively homosexual
○ Predominantly homosexual	○ Predominantly homosexual
○ Bisexual	○ Bisexual
○ Predominantly heterosexual	○ Predominantly heterosexual
○ Exclusively heterosexual	○ Exclusively heterosexual
○ Unsure	○ Unsure

In terms of comfort with my current sexual orientation, I would say that I am . . .

○ Very comfortable

○ Mostly comfortable

○ Comfortable

○ Not very comfortable

○ Very uncomfortable

TABLE 1. continued

INSTRUCTIONS:

Fill in the following circles by drawing lines to indicate which portion describes male or female elements. Indicate which portion of the circle is male by indicating (M) or female by indicating (F).

Example:

If the entire circle is male or female, simply indicate the appropriate symbol in the circle (M or F).

Example:

Fill out the circles indicating how it has been up to the present time as well as how you would like to see yourself in the future (ideal).

UP TO PRESENT TIME

Physical Identity
I was born as a biological...

Gender Identity
I think of myself as a physical...

In my sexual fantasies, I imagine myself as a physical...

Sex-Role Identity
My interests, attitudes, appearance and behaviors would be considered to be female or male (as traditionally defined)...

Sexual Orientation Identity
My sexual behavior has been with...

My sexual fantasies have been with...

My emotional attachments (not necessarily sexual) have been with...

FUTURE (IDEAL)

Physical Identity
Ideally, I wish I had been born as a biological...

Gender Identity
Ideally, I would like to think of myself as a physical...

In my sexual fantasies, I wish I could imagine myself as a physical...

Sex-Role Identity
I wish my interests, attitudes, appearance, and behaviors would be considered to be female or male (as traditionally defined)...

Sexual Orientation Identity
I wish my sexual behavior would be with...

I wish my sexual fantasies would be with...

I wish my emotional attachments (not necessarily sexual) would be with...

dimensions suggested by Shively and DeCecco [1977], [sexual behavior, fantasies and emotional attachments]). This opens up the broader perspective of ourselves as sexual beings or not simply defined by our genitalia.

Finally, the model assesses the ninth dimension to include the

136 CHEMICAL DEPENDENCY AND INTIMACY DYSFUNCTION

individual's past and present perceptions of their orientation and their idealized future. With this method, the problem of permanence of sexual orientation is addressed as well as yielding an additional measure of self acceptance.

The assessment device also allows for rating of past (including present) orientation as well as future or idealized orientations. This comparison gives the counselor and client some measure or indication of sexual orientation conflict or self acceptance. Obviously, the more discrepancies between dimensions, the more likelihood for lack of self-acceptance or discomfort with present functioning. Circle graphs are used rather than Kinsey (0 to 6) type ratings instead of individuals placing themselves on a line or adopting a certain number. Circles are used that individuals can divide into certain percentages or slices of a pie. The use of these circles seems to give the client a more graphic illustration of his or her sexual orientation in their natural complexity.

RECOMMENDATIONS

1. Counselors and treatment centers should develop a nonrestrictive definition of sexual health—one that allows for a variety of attitudes, beliefs, behaviors, and lifestyles. Unfortunately clients are often seen as less healthy based on the values and subjective judgments of the perceiver rather than objectively verifiable criteria. Staff of treatment centers need inservice training to examine their own attitudes concerning sexual health.
2. Staff members should explore their own sexuality and examine their possible biphobia and homophobia on an ongoing basis. (For a description of an inservice training program see Zigrang, 1982.)
3. Staff should be aware of heterosexual and monogamous biases and expectations and allow for more lifestyle alternatives.
4. Treatment centers should ensure that staff or consultants sensitive to sexual orientation issues are available to serve as resource persons and client role models.
5. Treatment centers should take time to inform guest speakers or resource people who work with their clients

about the kinds of appropriate language, exercises, discussion, etc. that do not discount alternative lifestyles and various sexual orientations.
6. It is important for counselors to initiate discussions of sexuality with clients. It is the professionals' responsibility to bring up the topic.
7. Counselors should help their clients explore their sexual orientation by:
   a. Asking direct questions.
   b. Constructing intake forms to offer options (heterosexual, lesbian/gay, bisexual, uncertain); the Klein Sexual Orientation Grid (Klein, 1980) or the Assessment Form developed by Coleman (1976) (See Table 1) should be utilized.
   c. Make sure forms, exercises and materials used in therapy or treatment accommodate alternative lifestyles.
   d. Incorporate into the lecture series information on sexual orientation.
   e. Add books on sexual orientation to the office library. Their presence is an invitation to talk about the issues.
8. If programs treating both men and women, offer general sexuality groups for women and men, the groups should be divided according to gender. At times, it can be useful to bring the groups together for discussion.
   a. Gender of facilitator should correspond to gender of group members. Whenever possible, a male and female co-therapist team can have some advantages.
   b. The entire range of sexuality and intimacy issues can and should be discussed in these groups.
   c. In the group, explore the aspects of sexual orientation. (See Table 1, for a worksheet for clients to complete.)
9. Develop a separate sexual orientation exploration group that would be optional for those clients who are gay/lesbian or bisexual or who are unsure of their sexual orientation.
   a. Help clients explore the relationship between their chemical use and sexual orientation.
   b. Help establish solidarity and support for chemically-free gay/lesbian or bisexual lifestyle.

c. Introduce gay/lesbian/bisexual staff who have attained sobriety to serve as role models.
10. Disclosure of sexual orientation needs to occur with discretion and respect for each person's unique life situation. It is helpful to be supportive but not demanding of the client in his or her attempt to come out either inside or outside of treatment.
11. If a client has disclosed his or her sexual orientation to his and her family, encourage open discussion and the processing of feelings about the client's sexual orientation.
12. Involve the partner or significant other of the gay/lesbian/or bisexual individual. The heterosexual bias of many treatment centers tends to avoid this or not push as hard for the involvement of others. These individuals need treatment and such treatment can increase the chances for rehabilitation of the chemically dependent individual. (See Whitney, 1982 and Colgan, 1987 for more descriptions of treating the co-alcoholic or the dependency patterns that so often develop.)
13. Encourage the clients to become involved with gay/lesbian or bisexual affiliated organizations.
14. Develop referral network for client aftercare needs including:
    a. Therapists who are openly identified as gay/lesbian/bisexual (see McNally and Finnegan, 1982).
    b. Therapists who are experienced in addressing sexuality/sexual identity issues.
    c. Sexual exploration groups.
    d. Lesbian/Gay/Bisexual AA/NA, Alanon and/or other twelve-step groups (Bittle, 1982).
15. Use tools for exploring sexuality such as a sexual orientation questionnaire (See Table 1).
16. Administrators and counselors should be aware of ways in which personnel sexually exploit clients both overtly and covertly. Confront such exploitation whenever you recognize it. This exploitation can take on several forms:
    a. Invasion of physical boundaries through inappropriate touch.
    b. Nontherapeutic use of sexual self-disclosure.

c. Therapeutic voyeurism of the client's sexual life.
d. Requiring the client to fit a heterosexual norm as a prerequisite to closure/graduation.

REFERENCES

Bales, R.F. (1946). Cultural differences in the rates of alcoholism. *Quarterly Journal of Studies on Alcohol, 6*, 480-499.
Beckman, L.J. (1979). Reported effects of alcohol on the sexual feelings and behavior of women alcoholics and non-alcoholics. *Journal of Studies on Alcoholism, 40*, 272-282.
Bittle, W.E. (1982). Alcoholics Anonymous and the Gay Alcoholic. *Journal of Homosexuality, 7*, 81-88.
Botwinick, J. and Machover, S. (1951). Psychometric examination of latent homosexuality in alcoholism. *Quarterly Journal of Studies on Alcoholism, 12*, 268-272.
Colcher, R.W. (1982). Counseling the homosexual alcoholic. *Journal of Homosexuality, 7*, 43-52.
Coleman, E. (1981-1982). Development stages of the coming out process. *Journal of Homosexuality, 7* (2/3), 31-43.
Coleman, E. (1987). Chemical dependency and intimacy dysfunction: Inextricably bound. *Journal of Chemical Dependency Treatment*, 1:1.
Coleman, E. (1987a). Assessment of Sexual Orientation. *Journal of Homosexuality*, in press.
Coleman, E. (1987b). Sexual compulsivity among chemically dependent individuals. *Journal of Chemical Dependency Treatment, 1*, in press.
Colgan, P. (1987). Treating dependency disorders in males: Toward a balance of identity and intimacy. *Journal of Chemical Dependency Treatment, 1*.
Covington, S.W. (1982). "Sex and Violence – The Unmentionable in Alcoholism Treatment." Paper presented at the National Alcoholism Forum of the National Council on Alcoholism, Washington, DC
DeCecco, J. Definition and meaning of sexual orientation. *Journal of Homosexuality, 9*(2/3), 1-26.
Fifield, L. (1975). *On My Way to Nowhere: Alienated, Isolated, Drunk*, Los Angeles: Gay Common Services Center.
Garfinkle, E. and Morin, S. (1978). Psychological attitudes toward homosexual psychotherapy clients. *Journal of Social Issues, 34*, 101-112.
Gibbins, R.J. and Walters, R.J. (1960). Three preliminary studies of a psychoanalytic theory of alcoholism. *Quarterly Journal of Studies on Alcohol, 21*, 618-641.
Gonsiorek, J. (1977). Psychological adjustment and homosexuality. *JSAS Catalog of Selected Documents, 7*, 45. (Ma.No. 1478).
Katz, J. (1976). *Gay American History: A Documentary of Lesbian and Gay Men in the U.S.A.* New York: Thomas Cromwell Co.
Kinsey, A.C., Pomeroy, W.B. and Martin, C.E. (1948). *Sexual Behavior in the Human Male*. Philadelphia: W.B. Saunders Co.
Kinsey, A.C., Pomeroy, W.B., Martin, C.E. and Gebhard, P.E. (1953). *Sexual Behavior in the Human Female*. Philadelphia: W.B. Saunders Co.
Klein, F. (1948). *The Bisexual Option*. New York: Arbor House Publishing Co.
Klein, F. (1980, December). Are you sure you're heterosexual? or homosexual? or even bisexual? *Forum Magazine*, pp. 41-45.

Lohrenz, L.J., Connelly, J.C., Coyne, L. and Spare, K. (1978). Alcohol problems in several mid-western homosexual communities. *Journal of Studies on Alcohol, 39*(11), 1959-1963.
McCord, W. and McCord, J. (1960). *Origins of Alcoholism.* Standford, CA: Stanford University Press.
McNally, E.M. and Finnegan, D.G. (1982). Working Together: The National Association of Gay Alcoholism Professionals, 7, 101-103.
Mongeon, J.E. and Ziebold, T.O. (1982). Preventing alcohol abuse in the gay community: Toward a theory and model. *Journal of Homosexuality, 7,* 89-99.
Nardi, P.M. (1982). Alcoholism and homosexuality: A theoretical perspective. *Journal of Homosexuality, 7,* 9-25.
Orlando (1978). Bisexuality: A choice Not an Echo. *Ms Magazine,* 7:(4), 60-75.
Prout, C., Strongin, E. and White, M. (1950). A Study of results in hospital treatment of alcoholism in males. *American Journal of Psychiatry, 107,* 14-19.
Quadland, M. (1985). Compulsive Sexual Behavior: Definition of a problem and an approach to treatment. *Journal of Sex and Marital Therapy, 11,* 121-132.
Saghir, M., Robins, E., Walbran, B. and Gentry, K. (1970). Homosexuality III: psychiatric disorders and disability in the female homosexual. *American Journal of Psychiatry, 127,* 147-154.
Schoener, G. (1976 January). The heterosexual norm in chemical dependency treatment programs: some personal observations. *Stock Capsules, 8.*
Shively, M. and DeCecco, J. (1977). Components of sexual identity. *Journal of Homosexuality, 3,* 41-48.
Small, E. and Leech, B. (1977). Counseling homosexual alcoholics: ten case histories. *Journal of Studies on Alcohol.* 38:(11), 2077-2086.
Smith, T.M. (1982). Specific approaches and techniques in the treatment of gay male alcohol abuses. *Journal of Homosexuality, 7,* 53-69.
Snyder, C. (1959). A Sociological View of the Etiology of Alcoholism in D.J. Pittman, ed. *Alcoholism: An Interdisciplinary Approach.* Springfield, IL: Charles C. Thomas Publishing Company.
Sterne, M., Schaefer, S. and Evans, S. (1983). Women's sexuality and alcoholism in P. Golding, ed., *Alcoholism: Analysis of a World-Wide Problem.* Lancaster, England: MTP Press Limited.
Swanson, D., Loomis, S., Lukesh, R., Cronin, R. & Smith, J. (1972). Clinical features of the female homosexual patient: a comparison with the heterosexual patient. *The Journal of Nervous and Mental Disease.* 155:(2), 119-124.
Weinberg, M. and Williams, C. (1974). *Male Homosexuals: Their Problems and Adaptations.* New York: Oxford University Press.
Whitney, S. (1982). The ties that bind: Strategies for Counseling the Gay Male Co-alcoholic. *Journal of Homosexuality, 7,* 37-41.
Ziebold, T. (1978). *Alcoholism and the Gay Community.* Washington, DC: Whitman-Walker Clinic and Blade Communications.
Ziebold, T. (1979 January). Alcoholism and Recovery: Gays helping gays. Christopher Street, pp. 36-44.
Zigrang, T.A. (1982). Who should be doing what about the gay alcoholic. *Journal of Homosexuality, 7,* 27-35.

Incest and Chemically Dependent Women: Treatment Implications

Sue Evans, MA
Susan Schaefer, MA

SUMMARY. This paper summarizes research which documents the correlation between chemical dependency and incest. It provides a conceptual framework for addressing incest on a continuum consisting of psychological precursors, covert incest and overt incest. The incest continuum which is described goes beyond mere legal definitions of incest and offers a definition of incest which the authors feel is more clinically meaningful and one which has implications for prevention, intervention, and treatment. This paper includes an assessment tool which the authors designed and have modified based on their clinical work and related research with incest victims. Recommendations for working with incest victims are outlined and an annotated bibliography is provided as a resource for both human service professionals and their clients who wish to explore the topic further.

Perhaps the earliest reference to the relationship between mood altering chemicals and incest can be traced to Genesis, in the story of Lot. This Biblical story (Genesis 19) serves as an excellent illustration of a number of dynamics common in inces-

---

Sue Evans is a certified chemical practitioner and AAECT-certified sex educator. Susan Schaefer is a licensed psychologist and certified chemical dependency practitioner.

Requests for reprints can be sent to Sue Evans at 2400 Blaisdell Avenue South, Minneapolis, MN 55404.

We would like to dedicate this paper to all the women and men who had the courage to share with us their struggles surrounding the impact of chemical dependency and incest in their lives and whose healing process we have been privileged to share. Special thanks to Judy Hoy and Patsy Foster for their work on the annotated bibliography.

© 1987 by The Haworth Press, Inc. All rights reserved.

tuous families: there is the obvious link with chemicals, as both Lot and his daughters were imbibing alcohol. Lot's wife had been transformed into a pillar of salt—a stark metaphor for frigidity or at the very least a statement of her withdrawal from her role as wife and mother. The daughters are implicated as responsible for getting Lot drunk and then initiating sex with him— clearly an example of blaming the victim, role reversal and blurring of generational lines—all common features in incestuous families.

While the relationship between chemical use/abuse and incest has been alluded to for centuries, systematic studies linking chemical dependency and incest have been published only recently beginning with the work of Benward and Densen-Gerber (1975). In a survey of a seven-state program for young women in recovery, Benward and Densen-Gerber found 44% of these 118 women they questioned acknowledged incest in their backgrounds.

Two years later, Ellen Weber (1977) reported in a study of 500 drug abusing adolescent females that 70% stated they had been sexually abused as children in their families.

Hammond, Jorgenson and Ridgeway (1979) reported 40% of the sample of chemically dependent women they surveyed had experienced incest in their past. They went on to note elevated rates of sexual dysfunction in this group of women.

With histories of both chemical dependency and incest, it could not be concluded from these studies that incest itself caused any greater sexual problems than otherwise might be expected given the significant influence chemical addiction itself has on sexual dysfunction.

However, by studying the differential rates of sexual dysfunction between two groups of alcoholic women—those who have histories of incest and those who do not—a better understanding of the impact of incest on later sexual difficulties can be ascertained. Hayek (1980) designed such a study and found the results clearly showed that the group of women who experienced incest were more likely to have started using chemicals sooner. They reported feeling much more uncomfortable during sex unless under the influence of chemicals and they showed higher incidence rates of vaginitis and dyspareunia.

In a study the authors conducted with Muriel Sterne (1983), 46% of the sample of 75 chemically dependent women stated they had experienced incest in their past. Thirteen percent of those who experienced incest were victimized by a female. Additionally, 13% admitted to their own sexual abuse of a minor. This research opened up an area little discussed or reported in prior research. This study indicated these events affected a significant proportion of women in recovery.

For many of these women their own acts of sexual abuse to minors often constitute the last bastion of shame for them in their recovery process, which, if left unaddressed, may threaten their sobriety.

Just as the literature has overlooked women as perpetrators of sexual abuse, so too has it often overlooked male victims. Father-son as well as mother-son incest needs to be further researched along with its specific relationship to chemical dependency. Anecdotal and unpublished reports of the incidence of incest among recovering males points to the need for further research. Dagney Christianson, Executive Director of Granville House, a chemical dependency halfway house in Minnesota, stated that one-quarter of the males questioned stated they had experienced incest in their childhoods when she first surveyed the residents (1979).[1]

While little research has focused on incest perpetrators and their involvement with chemicals, nonetheless, the few studies that have been published also point to a significant correlation between the use of mood altering chemicals and acts of incest. Virkkunen (1974) found in a study of 45 male perpetrators that 49% were alcoholic. Browning and Boatman (1977) reported over half the men involved in incest abused alcohol and Cavallin (1966) found one-third of the incestuous fathers "drank to an excess degree."

The relationship between chemical abuse and incest appears to be a significant one, warranting further study. From the onset, however, it is equally important to point out that not all perpetrators are chemically dependent or intoxicated at the time of their offenses, just as not all victims medicate their pain with chemicals or go on to become addicted. Moreover, for those perpetrators who are chemically dependent, termination of their chemical use does not always mark the end of their sexual offenses.

THE ROLE OF SOCIALIZATION

It is important to place this type of incest within the context of our socialization because it is not just an isolated problem. It is part of a larger social conditioning process involving sexism and female denigration. In this context, incest may be seen as simply one way in which the traditional model of male ownership of women and children manifested in this society.

There are, perhaps, few clearer examples of this sense of ownership than can be seen clinically in the typical incestuous family, where exaggerated sex roles are commonly observed. These male/female roles are often defined so rigidly that they appear to go beyond mere stereotypes and become caricatures of the male and female roles prescribed by the larger society, where men predominantly hold the positions of power. In incestuous families, the line of power is often clearly defined as moving from father to son(s), then to mother and finally to daughter(s) rather than from parent to child. This necessarily creates an hierarchy which, by its very nature blurs generational lines of authority. This produces an atmosphere ripe for the emergence of role-reversal (children taking on adult responsibilities while parents abdicate their role), codependency (unhealthy caretaking behavior) and unmet dependency needs of the children (of which more will be said later). These power dynamics produce patterns which promote an atmosphere in which intimacy needs are met in dysfunctional ways within the family.

Rigid sex role conditioning may also account for some of the differences observed between male and female victims, but such differences tend to parallel the traditional sex role training of this culture. The socialization process has traditionally taught females to be passive, submissive caretakers, who suffer from unrestrained emotionality which they are taught to internalize in self defeating ways (Butler, 1978).

Wilsnack (1973) has noted the connection between women's chemical use and attempts to compensate for feelings of sex role inadequacy. This sexual socialization polarizes women into virgin/whore or frigid/promiscuous roles, offering no latitude for a healthy model of female sexuality. Women are taught that power lies outside themselves and is accessible only through males. Sex for many women is one of the few barter tools they know can be used to access this power. Clearly, this is "victim training."

Males on the other hand, are traditionally taught to be active, decisive, aggressive, unemotional; trained to act out their pain in externalized ways. (Noted in the higher rates of auto fatalities, homicides and other violent crimes.) With respect to sexuality, they are expected to be the seekers and conquerors, ever ready to perform sexually or to be thought unmasculine. Clearly, when carried to the extreme—"victimizer training." Traditional sex role conditioning may explain why there appears to be proportionately more male victims who become perpetrators than females from these incestuous families.

There exists greater social approval for males to learn about sex experimentally and to be given more latitude in which to express themselves sexually without being labelled negatively. This certainly has a positive effect, in that males do not have to suffer from the virgin/whore syndrome as do females, but it also has a negative effect in the cultural failure to notice male victimization. The recent trend in American motion picture films depicting teenage boys "learning about sex" or "having their greatest dreams come true" with older women ("Class," "Risky Business," and "My Tutor") points to this phenomenon. The boys are depicted as being lucky and fulfilled—certainly not victims. The reality is that adults having sex with minors legally constitutes child abuse. Currently all states now have child abuse laws requiring the reporting of sexual abuse.

When males experience incest then, it is often more difficult for them to label it as abusive and to see themselves as victims. Many may feel confused but report little trauma. Others may feel queasy and wonder, "What's wrong with me? I should be enjoying this and I'm not." Females, on the other hand, are more apt to experience incest as abuse and ask "What's wrong with me? What did I do to cause this?" They are also ten times more likely to absorb the guilt.[2]

The social failure to recognize male sexual abuse may, in part, account for the lower reported rates of male incest victims. While we believe that overt female incest is still higher than is true for males, there exists a need for improved identification of male victims and a rethinking of male sex-role expectations to arrive at more accurate, and perhaps similar, rates of incest.

The socialization process trains; female children to be victims, male children to be victimizers, and sanctions incest by ignoring the problem, and continues the process by making new victimizers out of old victims.

INCEST AS AN INTERGENERATIONAL PHENOMENON

Incest does not occur in a vacuum. It has been found to be multigenerational (Rosenfeld, Nadelson, Krieger & Backman, 1977; Summit & Kryso, 1978) in nature, that is, it is passed on from one generation to another through the family roles and rules. Rules regarding touch/nontouch, affection and intimacy expression, privacy and respect for personal boundaries are all important in the development of incestuous behavior. Much like alcoholism, which can also be traced intergenerationally, incest may appear to skip a generation. With alcoholism this often takes the form of a generation of "teetotalers" interspersed between two generations of active alcoholics. So too, can it appear that incest skips generations. Sometimes in an effort to insure that they will not be sexually inappropriate with their child (as may have been true in their own history), parents may withhold touch out of their own fear of not being able to touch safely. While not active sexual abuse, the child pays a high price for the unresolved incestuous fears governing the parent. This can become a set up for the child to seek touch in any way possible — leaving the child more vulnerable to outside sexual abuse because their touch needs have not been met. It also sets up the child to seek out touch inappropriately because of tremendous unmet touch needs.

BOUNDARY FORMATION

Boundaries might best be viewed as the physical and psychic space around us. Families as well as cultures vary in their established rules regarding appropriate boundaries (comfort zone between two persons standing, eye gaze intensity, affectionate touch displayed in public, etc.). It is the task of parents to teach appropriate boundaries, much like any other basic learning. Through this process a child learns s/he is a separate individual with individual rights (Kaplan, 1978). She/he learns the joy of making decisions, mastery over developmental tasks, how to be trusted as well as trust for others, and a perception of the world as safe or threatening. Included in this basic learning about boundaries are such things as: (1) how to maintain confidences; (2) knocking before entering closed doors; (3) respect of personal belongings; (4) privacy for mail and diaries; (5) and respectful touch.

When boundaries are violated by emotional, physical or sexual intrusions it is as if someone rips open the victim, reaches in and "steals their soul." In later relationships, they often experience a terror of being "swallowed up" and losing their sense of self for they have learned that closeness/touch "takes away" rather than "gives" to them. This struggle to protect themselves from intimacy feels like a life/death struggle for survival. Requests are seen as demands by these persons, closeness is perceived as losing oneself, and affection puts one in touch with the "empty gaping hole" inside: the "hole" that carries all the unmet childhood needs; for many experienced as a hollow bottomless pit of neglect and despair.

For many there is also a strong fear of abandonment that is operating concurrently with the fear of intimacy. This fear of abandonment motivates the person to reach out for relationships while at the same time the fear of intimacy may cause them to withdraw resulting in an approach/avoidance dance that can be very confusing to partners.

These boundary problems are the basis of intimacy dysfunction, which has been highly correlated to individuals with chemical dependency (Coleman, 1982). Comparisons made between chemically dependent and non-chemically dependent individuals have shown that the chemically dependent individuals have experienced more "boundary inadequacy" in growing up (Coleman & Colgan, 1986).

Emotional Boundary Violations

Boundaries are learned and in early childhood often require a given stage of neural and muscular development to perform. At birth, it is as if the infant is one with the parent. A symbiotic relationship develops between the primary care giver (usually the mother) and the child—each giving the other fulfillment. As the baby develops neurologically its senses are better able to establish it as separate from its parent (Kopp, 1980). This separation task is also one the parent needs to perform concurrently with the child. If the parent has difficulty with this letting go process for some reason, boundary problems often arise. The parent's possessiveness, insecurity, shame or narcissism can all contribute to an interference with this individuation process. A common result is for the child to only feel valued for what s/he can give to the parent. This begins the process of role-reversal, whereby the child assumes adult responsibilities for the parent, so common in incestuous and chemically dependent families.

If the parent is insecure about her/himself, an expectation may develop that the child be perfect—clean at all times, smiling throughout all visits with relatives and able to perform great feats to entertain others (Miller, 1981). When the child acts out, it may tap the parent's feeling of shame and worthlessness. As long as the child can be controlled the parent is better able to maintain a sense of adequacy.

Other examples of emotional boundary violations may be seen in rigid feeding or toilet training schedules (expecting the child to be toilet trained before s/he is physiologically capable of the task, thus setting the child up for failure), listening in on phone conversations, or making all decisions for the child regarding clothing, friends, choice of social activities, expecting to be told all the personal thoughts and experiences of the child, etc. These emotional boundary violations teach the child that her/his value is in caretaking others (Hammer, 1976). As a result, basic dependency needs of the child often go unmet.

As the child grows older s/he may be restricted from contacts with persons outside the family (Weinberg, 1976). Rigid, nonpermeable boundaries are often set up around incestuous families, insulating the family from the rest of the world. Sometimes enmeshed parents are jealous and threatened at their child's attempts to form friendships. To control these efforts, parents may criticize their children's efforts at making friends by citing flaws in these prospective companions. Then, too, the children themselves may curtail their own activities with others — especially bringing friends into their house — due to their sense of fear or shame surrounding the incest. Family cohesion revolves around maintaining the secret, consciously or unconsciously. With these rigid boundaries built into the structure of incestuous families, a further harmful consequence is the lack of reality testing available to family members, who may go on for years believing most families operate similarly to their own.

Physical Boundary Violations

Physical violations are a second primary area in which boundaries may be invaded. Holding a child down against her/his will, continued tickling to and beyond the point of pain, or poking at parts of the child's body (ears, navel, etc.) are all examples of physical boundary violations. More extreme examples are hitting or beating. In all cases, the message is clear that the child does not own her/his body and there is no safety from unwanted physical intrusions.

Sexual Boundary Violations

Sexual abuse is a third primary area in which boundary violations may take place. These sexual abuses may be covert (camouflaged) or overt (blatant). What accounts for the manner in which some family members violate sexual boundaries, if at all, or do so covertly instead of overtly, can only be speculated on. The perpetrator's own history, the parental relationship/bond, strong religious convictions, or fear of reprisal may in part account for differences in these patterns.

DEFINITIONS OF INCEST

Legal definitions of what constitutes incestuous behavior typically require the presence of (1) blood related parties, and where (2) intercourse has occurred.[3] Therapeutically, it is important to expand definitions of incest to include a broader framework: One which incorporates the psychological dynamics which set the stage for incest to occur, as well as ambiguous behaviors where an intended or felt sexual connotation is present; on through more blatant sexual behaviors to include sexual contact as well as penetration. For this reason, incest might best be viewed conceptually along a continuum consisting of psychological, covert and overt incest. See Table 1.

Overt Incest

We feel that incest is present whenever sexual contact or penetration occurs between any two members of a primary family grouping (as opposed to blood relatives only). This allows for the inclusion of stepparents, stepbrothers or sisters, as well as lovers of the parents who may or may not be living in the home. Sexual contact should include both direct touch and indirect touch (i.e., through clothing) of sexual body parts. Penetration broadens no-

Table 1

Incest Continuum

Psychological Precursors	Covert	Overt
Enmeshment/Disengagement	"Inadvertent Touch"	French Kissing
Blurring of Generational Lines	Household Voyeurism	Fondling
	Sexualizing Remarks	Cunnilingus
Role Reversal	Ridicule of Developing Body	Fellatio
Unmet Dependency Needs		Intercourse
Touch Deprivation	Viewing or Reading of Pornographic Materials (Parent to Child)	Sodomy
Shame-based Family System		Penetration with Objects
Disrespected Privacy Needs		Exhibitionism
	Overly Strict Household Dress Codes	
	Sexual Hugs	

tions of intercourse to include intrusions of any type, (i.e., finger or objects as well as penis to vagina intercourse).

Case Study 1 – Pam

Pam entered therapy at a time when she was experiencing nightmares related to her childhood incest experiences. She had been waking up from her own screams at night as she relived in her dreams some of her past sexual abuse. She reported feeling generally very unsafe, even in her own home. Over the past months she had felt very vulnerable and had withdrawn from those persons closest to her, unable to get support. Recently, she had become very self-abusive, cutting her arms with a razor on several occasions.

Pam stated that she was 2 years into her "recovery" from alcoholism. She traced the origins of her first drinking to attempts to ease her fears as she was first experiencing sexual relationships with boys in high school. Once out of high school, Pam stated she "sexually acted out a lot" during her periods of heaviest drinking. Once "sober," she found she had many fears over being sexual which remained unresolved.

Pam's Family History. For most of Pam's younger years, Pam's mother was chronically ill and had been addicted to tranquilizers. As the oldest daughter, Pam was expected to take over many of the household chores, as well as caring for her four younger siblings.

Prior to her mother's illness, Pam and her father developed a close bond. Pam's father had a poor relationship with his wife and used to complain to Pam about his marital problems. As time went on, Pam's father received most of his emotional needs through Pam, as he increasingly turned to her for companionship and physical comforting. By the time Pam was 7, he also began meeting his sexual needs through her by kissing and genital touching. When Pam was 9, she spent a weekend with her maternal grandparents during which time her grandfather fondled her also.

At age 13, having been sexual with her father over a 6 year period of time, her father suddenly seemed to lose interest in her and started being sexual with Pam's younger sister, age 6. While it was a great relief for her to not have to satisfy his sexual needs, she also experienced great emotional difficulty as his attention shifted. She felt very threatened by her sister, jealous and left out from her father's attention, and resentful about losing her special place in the family.

She told her mother about both her father's and her grandfather's sexual activities with her, but her mother didn't believe her and punished her for lying. She told a priest about the incest and he recommended she pray, stating that he couldn't do anything to stop the abuse because it was important the family stay together.

Pam reported a childhood sexual history which included being sexual with cousins, little friends, and older boys. As an adolescent, she experienced a neighbor exposing himself to her and in her senior year was raped by one of her teachers.

Feeling frustrated and alone, Pam turned to alcohol to medicate her pain. Her use of alcohol became habitual and began to seriously interfere with interpersonal functioning. She began to experience hallucinations and disassociations and ultimately became suicidal. Pam eventually entered chemical dependency treatment as her alcoholism worsened.

This is a fairly typical example of overt incest between father and daughter. In most cases of overt abuse, there are some covert and psychological violations occurring as well. In this case, the father was looking to the child to fulfill the marital bond that was lacking with his wife.

In Pam's case, her Mother's denial allowed the abuse to continue, thereby not giving Pam or her sister the protection they needed. In other cases, parents immediately report the offending father and remove the child to safety, but this is not the typical scenario.

The psychic/sexual bond between the incest father and his daughter puts a terrible strain on the child but also gives them special power within the family. "Incest envy" is a term the authors don't use. However, it refers to a concept important to address. The "chosen" child might get special attention from an otherwise neglectful parent(s) (i.e., special privileges or even money to bribe her/him to secrecy). The other sibling and spouse often resent the "chosen" one since in neglected families there is the myth of finite love—the belief that there is not enough love to go around and if one child receives it the others will starve emotionally.

The parent who, like Pam's father, consistently picks children from a specific age group to get her/his needs met is often operating at an immature psychosexual level. It is as if the parent is fixated at an earlier developmental age and is attempting to find partners that aren't threatening.

Pam was more vulnerable to other forms of abuse because she was not taught appropriate boundaries or ways of taking proper care of herself. It is quite common for victims to feel that they are to blame for the violations and to seek out some form of punishment to atone for this guilt. Self punishment can occur on many levels. Consistently putting themselves into abusive relationships (because it feels so familiar), self mutilation or simply not taking care of themselves are typical ways victims punish themselves.

The hallucinations and disassociations Pam experienced often begin as psychological defenses employed by incest victims usually (initially at least) during the actual sexual abuse. In order to withstand the trauma of what for many involves chronic acts of abuse, some victims mentally disassociate. For some, this is described as "merging with the wall." For others it involves mentally escaping their body and viewing the abuse as a spectator from above. For still others, who have experienced a combination of chronic physical and sexual abuse, this level of disassociation can escalate to the mental creation of a new personality withstanding the abuse (i.e., multiple personality). Once out of their families, victims may continue to experience the sensory dysperceptions and disassociations, especially, during periods of stress or threat to their safety. Later, as adults, many victims report an extensive history of psychiatric interventions (psychotherapy, shock treatment, hospitalization) aimed at treating the very emotional and behavioral survival mechanisms which once helped them cope with the abuse but then go on to haunt them uncontrollably.

Taking on the victim role is probably one of the more damaging ways victims are affected by incest. This goes beyond merely being violated. It includes assuming a whole set of attitudes and behaviors and perceiving oneself as a victim in all that one does. It involves a negative, fatalistic mind-set, a belief that a price will be exacted for anything good that happens, and the perception of powerlessness acted out in what often appears to be a chronic, paralyzing learned helplessness. Long after the violations stop this victim role may continue on.

Covert Incest

Covert incest carries many of the same dynamics as overt incest, shrouded with an added element of confusion. Covert incest is present when psychological dynamics combine with behaviors which carry a purposeful (perpetrator) or felt (victim) sexual connotation. Among a variety of covert incestuous behaviors are the following:

1. *Inadvertent Touch* — touch which under the guise of some other explicit set of behaviors includes an implicit sexual intent. For example: A father wrestles with his daughter and regularly brushes against her breasts consciously, while pretending his actions are accidental.
2. *Household Voyeurism* — lascivious gazing at a family member and being disrespectful of privacy needs are key elements to this form of violation. Examples include peeping through key holes or drilling holes through walls to view members naked or conducting private activities.
3. *Sexualizing Remarks* — any remark designed to objectify a child. Examples include calling an adolescent female a slut/whore or describing a child as seductive, thereby imputing an adult sexual motive onto the child.
4. *Ridicule of Developing Body* — another form of sexualizing a child. Adolescence is a difficult time regarding body image anyway, without added shaming or ridiculing. Example: A young woman woke up one morning to find her brother had put bandaids on her nipples and several family members were around her bed laughing at her small breasts.
5. *Viewing or Reading Pornographic Materials with a Child* — this describes an adult to child collegial relationship which blurs appropriate generational lines and adds another damaging element — teaching children about sex in ways which typically promote the subordination and denigration of

women. Example: A father uses a pornographic film he has rented to teach his adolescent son about sex.
6. *Overly Strict Household Dress Codes* — dress codes which carry an implicit sexual message — don't wear this because it sexually arouses someone in the family. Example: A mother cautions her adolescent daughter not to wear her pajamas or swimsuit around her father, thus making the child responsible for the adult's sexuality.
7. *Sexual Hugs* — Hugs which take away from the child by arousing or satisfying the sexual needs of the parent.

Case Study 2 — Mary

Mary entered therapy because she had had a pattern of abusive relationships with men that she wanted to change. She was afraid of touch because affectionate touch always became confused with sexual touch for her, leaving her feeling out of control and powerless. She was afraid of intimacy on any level unless it was with an emotionally sick or alcoholic man with whom she could feel a strength gained from her efforts to change or rescue him.

Mary's Family History. Mary's mother was a kindly, passive, self-effacing woman who readily accepted blame for most everything wrong in her world. She obsessed over even the smallest of mistakes, often making repeated apologies for ones made years ago.

Mary's father was a dominant and angry man, uninvolved emotionally with her family. The children feared him and kept much of their life hidden from him. Mary's mother served as "protector" and would frequently argue with him over differences in parenting the children. These arguments made Mary feel guilty and responsible.

Mary had three siblings, a brother and two sisters, all several years older than Mary. Clearly, the males held greater power in the family. They made all major decisions, were waited on, and received special privileges and attention.

The family rules were such that rights of privacy were ignored. Mary reported frequently dressing in the closet as she was afraid someone would walk in on her, and when in the bathroom she would always prop one foot against the door.

Mary had no memory of being molested, yet she remembered being fearful that her brother had wanted to be sexual with her. He had never talked about being sexual with her, however, she remembers him showing her one of his pornographic magazines. Mary's fears of her brother confused her since it appeared to her to have developed out of nowhere to her. Despite this fear, Mary continued to look up to her brother as a role model and valued their relationship. He had been much like a father to her — making sure she got to bed on time, brushing her hair, wrestling with her, and reading stories to her. At times Mary chastised herself for having these concerns about her brother because they seemed unfounded.

Mary began sex play with her friends when she was six. They played a game in which one of the participants pretended she was forceful and aggressive while the other would struggle and say "No, no, don't do that."

Mary began having sexual intercourse at age 13 with males 18-20 years old. She stated she always felt older and in charge of this decision, and resisted the suggestion that these relationships were abusive. She continued on through her adult life picking men who were dependent on her emotionally, yet would abuse her physically.

Mary later learned from a sister that her older brother had forced sex on her two sisters when Mary was a very young child.

This is an example of covert incest dynamics between Mary and her brother. Even though she had never (to her knowledge) been molested by her brother, Mary was still greatly affected by the family system in which incest had occurred.

Covert incest is often more difficult to deal with than overt incest because there is no concrete incident to base the feelings of violation. Therefore the victim assumes it is only her/his own "craziness."

The amount of trauma associated with sibling incest seems to be dependent upon the power imbalance rather than the actual sex act. Siblings of about the same age or the same power (note: males hold more power within each age group, so even if the age matches, the power might still be imbalanced) could conceivably be sexual with little damage to the participants. In fact, some women have reported that their families were so dysfunctional that the closeness and intimacy gained in a sexual relationship with a close sibling helped them survive — clearly a sad commentary on their neglected dependency needs.

As the age and power differential increases so does the emotional trauma. This speaks to the issue of incest being primarily an issue of power, acted out in a sexual arena rather than a sexual problem *per se*.

PSYCHOLOGICAL PRECURSORS OF INCEST

The psychological underpinnings which are present in incestuous families are likely to include a number of dysfunctional family dynamics which not only make possible, but, one could argue, make probable covert or overt expressions of sexuality within the family. Among these psychological underpinnings may be found the following:

1. *Enmeshment* — families where little outside input is allowed. The family is often overprotected from outsiders and under-protected from insiders. Developmental separation and individuation is usually fought by the parents every step of the way. Family members are expected to meet most of the needs of each other, routinely reinforced by outsiders being rejected by other family members. In conjunction with the enmeshment, disengagement patterns are commonly observed in incestuous families where family members isolate from each other in order to feel separateness. This isolation continues, often times until there is a crisis which brings family members running to the rescue. A pseudo-intimacy is then set up reinforcing crisis-oriented behavior as a means to get one's needs met.
2. *Blurring of Generational Lines* — a defined childhood status is often lacking as children are expected to assume a maturity well in advance of their years. With this expectation parents often relate to them more like a colleague, peer or

spouse, exposing emotional vulnerabilities, sharing with them the burdens of the provider role, or expecting them to provide the social intimacies they need—such as talking to the child about their intimate sexual problems.
3. *Role Reversal*—takes the above dynamic one step further with children assuming a primary care-giver role to either parent (especially where alcoholism, drug addiction, physical or psychological illness is involved) or to younger siblings when parents abdicate their role.
4. *Unmet Dependency Needs*—when children are expected, at too early age, to adopt adult responsibilities, their lives as children are necessarily cut short. With this, a number of their own dependency needs go unmet. For some, this takes the form of neglect where basic physical or emotional needs go unmet. For others, it is experienced in physical or sexual abuse where important safety needs are not met.
5. *Touch Deprivation*—one basic human need is the need for touch—touch that gives affection without reference to ulterior motives—touch that is warm and spontaneous. When the need for touch is not met infants are known to have emotional, physical or intellectual impairments, or even to die—a condition referred to as marasmus.
6. *Shame*—Perhaps singularly so, shame stands out as the primary emotion experienced in incestuous families. It is the funnel through which nearly all other felt emotions get translated. The origin of shame (see Kaufman, 1980) seems clearly linked to the unmet dependency needs of a child, who in her/his own egocentric rationalizations believes that if her/his parents aren't giving as they should, it must be because s/he is unworthy of these gifts. The sense of unworthiness, more than anything else, when repeated over time forms the basis of a shame-based identity, so predominant in individuals coming from an incestuous family. Additionally, there is often very active shaming going on by family members to each other. This system is based on a shame/blame cycle, where the family looks to see who is to blame rather than how to solve the problem.
7. *Disrespected Privacy Needs*—involves violations of emotional and physical boundaries and space.

Case Study 3 – Jane

Jane came to therapy with presenting complaints of anxiety and depression. Throughout the course of her therapy Jane struggled with unclear boundaries and codependency (unhealthy caretaking behavior) in a number of areas of her life. She experienced an immense amount of guilt and shame, taking on responsibility for anything that went wrong around her. This caretaker role led her to take on numerous causes of social injustice, often at her own expense.

In relationships, Jane frequently experienced other's pain as her own and felt compelled to "fix it." She became frightened if others wanted to be close to her unless she could act the caretaker. Once she let herself trust and be close to someone, she developed a hostile-dependency in that relationships, burying her rage. Lacking a clear sense of her own boundaries in relation to others, Jane found herself oscillating between enmeshment and disengagement in her relationships.

Jane's Family History. Jane shared a special relationship with her mother, who felt especially bonded to Jane as if they were "buddies" or equals. Jane's Dad was alcoholic, authoritarian and absent from home especially when serving in the military. When he came home, he got drunk and physically abusive. Jane's mother would, at times, sleep with Jane for protection, comfort and solace. She frequently confided in Jane her secret dreams, discussed the abusive relationship she had with Jane's father, and shared her sexual frustrations. During her parent's arguments, Jane always felt in the middle and found herself resorting to many tactics to get them to stop. If they continued fighting or drinking, Jane felt like a failure. To escape her family's pain, Jane often immersed herself in her schoolwork and extracurricular activities, appearing as a model student.

This is an example of psychological boundary violations. In order for Jane to have gotten any of her needs met, she first needed to attend to her mother's needs. This, in effect, resulted in her feeling shamed for being "needy." Her job was to "caretake" her mother, not to be a child with childlike needs. Jane coped with this by working hard to be successful. Not all incest victims fit the typical victim role. Some have learned to mask their inner insecurity, appearing quite competent. Others assume a pseudo-maturity. Still others become perfectionists, working desperately to be in control of some aspect of their lives (external) in order to feel more in control of their feelings (internal). Victims often become very controlling of other people and situations. Their very safety once depended upon learning how to read others emotionally and learning to control them either overtly or passively.

Internally, however, they report feeling shameful, scared, tentative, helpless, and chameleon-like, adjusting themselves to fit appropriately with whomever they are with, in the hope of being accepted.

We would not label Jane as incest victim (nor anyone who just experienced psychological violations), but rather she is a victim of boundary violations and is an adult child of an alcoholic. However, many of her therapy issues overlap with those of an incest victim.

INCEST ASSESSMENT

How each person manifests symptoms of incest varies, with some people choosing more internalized modes of expression while others will show a more externalized expression of their symptoms. While it is unlikely that any person would exhibit all symptoms correlated to incest, nonetheless a pattern of symptoms typically will emerge for victims of covert or overt incest.[5] Insofar as this is true, the authors have developed the following assessment form:

I. BEHAVIORAL CUES FOR THE DIAGNOSIS OF INCEST

Incest victims frequently act out their pain in a variety of seriously self-abusive ways, as if to acknowledge overtly the pain they are experiencing and achieve some congruity between their insides (feelings) and their outsides (that part visible to others). Among those persons where incest has not yet been diagnosed, the following behavior patterns often emerge where overt/covert

incest is eventually determined (rarely would an individual experience all symptoms):
A. Chemical Abuse/Dependency
B. Self-Mutilating Behaviors
  1. Cutting or carving patterns in the skin
  2. Burning
  3. Hitting self
  4. Punching out windows or walls
  5. Pulling hair out
  6. Self tatooing
C. Eating Disorders
  1. Overeating
  2. Anorexia
  3. Bulimia
D. Suicide Attempts
E. Truancy, Learning Problems
F. Delinquency, Running Away from Home
G. Isolation and Inability to Relate to Peers
H. Sexual Knowledge and Sophistication Well Beyond Age Appropriateness
I. Sexual Dysphoria
  1. Disinterest
  2. Fears/Phobias
  3. Disgust
J. Sexual Dysfunction
  1. Vaginismus
  2. Dispareunia
  3. Inhibited sexual desire
K. Sexual Acting Out
  1. Compulsive sexual behavior/Sex addiction
  2. Seductive behavior (manipulative sexual behavior)
  3. Selling of sex-prostitution, stripping, pornography
  4. Sexual offenses
L. Sexual Self-Abuse
  1. Attempts to desexualize self
    a. obvious attempts to hide behind clothes
    b. binding breasts or genitals
    c. cutting or harming sexual body parts

2. Involvement in sado-masochistic sexual behaviors with harmful consequences.
M. Sleeping Disorders
   1. Recurrent attack nightmares
   2. Fear of falling asleep
   3. Sleep walking
   4. Light sleep with frequent startle responses
N. Physiological Symptoms
   1. Gastrointestinal: colitis, ulcers, lower abdominal pain
   2. Gynecological: frequent infection, pain with intercourse, menstrual difficulties
O. General Victim Behavior
   1. Passivity
   2. Behavior which provokes others and sets one up for attack
   3. Failure to protect or take care of oneself properly
   4. Overwillingness to accept blame
   5. Pattern of abusive relationships
   6. Learned helplessness
P. Fear of Intimacy
   1. Approach-avoidance in relationships
   2. Feelings of being overwhelmed, losing self in relationships
   3. Chronic enmeshment/disengagement pattern
Q. Fear of Touch/Touch Deprivation
R. Caretaking Behavior/Maturity Beyond Age Appropriateness
S. Role Reversal
   1. Assuming parental responsibilities
   2. Feeling responsible for parent's feelings and behaviors
   3. Protecting parents — covering up for them
T. Perfectionism

II. PSYCHOLOGICAL CUES FOR THE DIAGNOSIS OF INCEST

While many people experience the following feelings, particularly the more general ones, the distinction in assessing incest victims involves the intensity and chronicity of the emotions.

Incest victims typically incorporate these generalized emotions into a protective posture, using these emotions as defensive strategies or coping mechanisms—often consciously—to survive. They then become integrated into their general personality structure (trait) as opposed to their being expressed merely as a response to a specific experience (state).

A. Shame
B. Guilt
C. Self-Hatred
D. Depression
E. Anxiety/Phobias
F. Grief and Loss Issues
G. Low Self-Esteem, Feelings of Worthlessness
H. Guardedness—Inability to Trust; Secrecy and Withdrawal
I. Dramatic Personality Changes
J. Boundary Ambiguity
   1. Identity diffusion—no clear sense of self
   2. Enmeshment/disengagement
K. Very large or extremely small psychic/spacial needs
L. Disassociative/surfacy behavior—difficulty concentrating, a sense of detachment from one's body—a feeling of not really being present.
M. Sensory dysperceptions, hallucinations
N. Flashbacks

III. COVERT FAMILIAL CUES:
DID ANYONE IN YOUR FAMILY EVER . . .

A. Try to seduce your young friends?
B. Tell dirty stores, view pornographic magazines or movies with you?
C. Ridicule your developing body?
D. Repeatedly make accusations or punish you for being sexual when it wasn't true?
E. Physically punish you while naked or force you to strip clothing before receiving the punishment?
F. Ask questions or share explicit details regarding his/her sex life?

G. Engage in "Inadvertent" sexual touch?
H. Sleep with you when they were feeling needy?
I. Fail to respect requests for privacy while dressing, in the bathroom, or at other times when you did not want intrusion?
J. Ask you to not be seen around the house in pajamas, bathing suit or other attire which may suggest uncomfortableness with your body?
K. Gaze at you in ways you felt were sexual glances?
L. Have you ever been afraid someone in your family wanted to/would become sexual with you?

RECOMMENDATIONS

1. In order to provide professional treatment of the issue of incest or family sexual abuse among chemically dependent individuals and their families, the clinician needs specialized education (beyond therapeutic skills) in the areas of sexual family abuse, victim behavior, family systems theory, and boundary development.

2. The clinician needs ongoing group supervision or a good clinical supervisor knowledgeable in this area to assist the clinician in keeping track of the transference/counter transference issues. This helps keep the system open, as it is very easy to become enmeshed into the client's family system.

3. The clinician needs a good referral and support network of other professionals who work with victims/victimizers as these clients often require adjunctive therapy (chemical dependency treatment, psychiatric medication/hospitalization, bulimia/anorexia treatment, etc.).

4. The clinician needs a basic understanding and utilization of feminist therapy as it is extremely helpful and necessary to place the familial abuse within the context of the larger social structure.

5. It is necessary to maintain a high level of self-care. The therapeutic process of working with victims is very seductive. To become the "saviour," the only one who can help the client, is a particular trap for clinicians who are often overworked and overstressed.

a. Maintain personal relationships/life.
b. Balance emotional, physical, intellectual, sexual and spiritual needs so as to not be tempted to fulfill them through the client.

6. It is crucial not to contribute to the damage. Counter transference issues are easily triggered. If client's issues trigger clinician's past abuse or family history it is important to get therapeutic help to deal directly with these issues rather than working them out through the client.

7. It is important to take advantage of educational opportunities in that new understandings are being developed every day as this is a relatively new field.

SUGGESTIONS FOR WORKING WITH CLIENTS

The authors realize the importance of family systems theory and working to evoke change in the whole family, but these recommendations are limited in scope to the individual therapeutic process.

1. It is crucial to maintain firm boundary setting with clients. As a clinician, you need it to survive professionally as well as to model good boundary setting for clients, as it helps them to feel safe. You teach boundary setting by having boundaries. Some specific ways of setting boundaries include:
   a. Don't allow calls at home.
   b. Be very clear that you are not going to be their friend, socialize with them, or sexualize the relationship.
   c. Be cautious in responding to their crises with extra appointments, special care, etc. This keeps them in a crisis mode of getting their needs met.
   d. Limit self-disclosure to appropriate levels. Self-disclosure should only be used when it's intent is to broaden or deepen the client's understanding of themselves.
   e. Don't allow them to be mean or abusive to you. You will then become a part of their system, and untrustable. It is important to role model someone who takes care of themselves.
   f. If you are seeing the individual in group psychotherapy,

have clear and unambiguous rules in the group that everyone agrees to. These rules would include:
- No sexual contact can be allowed between group members.
- Start and end group promptly. Example: If you run over time because one person is in crisis, the rest of the group might feel a need to compete for extra time/special attention also.
- Hold clients accountable for homework assignments/ payment. If you do not hold them accountable, you give the message that they are helpless, not able to take care of themselves, or are not adults.

g. Ask for permission about touch or nurturing them. Keep in mind that touch has been abusive. By respecting their physical boundaries you teach boundary setting.

2. It's helpful to eventually work in a group setting to end the client's feeling of isolation set up by keeping the secret (family roles). It is important to have a co-therapist for this group as it is easy to feel overwhelmed and assume the hopelessness and despair of the clients. Co-therapists can better circumvent this. (By operating within the context of the Incest Continuum, the authors put both covert and overt victims of incest in the same group.)

3. It is helpful to assess and stabilize any biochemical imbalances before addressing deep rooted emotional issues. Also, utilize psychometric testing to assess for ego strength and the possible need for medication.

4. Reframe the self-destructive behaviors that brought them into therapy. The Incest Assessment form is helpful in putting each individual client's behavior into the context of the common survival skills of victims. This is helpful in lessening their feelings of shame. Address those behaviors as ways they have tried to deal with the pain of the abuse, but now those defenses are getting in the way of their "recovery." Increase their repertoire of constructive survival skills (i.e., telling the secrets, expressing the feelings — especially anger, self-care, getting support from other people, etc.) rather than forcing them to give up their favorite defenses.

5. Explore abuse within the context of the continuum frame-

work (previously described), validating psychological and covert as well as overt forms of abuse.

6. It's important to not attempt in-depth therapy when they are still actively abusing themselves (i.e., chemical abuse, cutting their bodies, bulimia, involved in an abusive relationship, etc.). It is often necessary to stabilize these abusive behaviors first. The authors regularly suggest abstinence from any chemical use (even for those who are not chemically dependent) while in the therapeutic process so as to not medicate their feelings.

7. Gently point out any victim behavior you see in your relationship with them, in group or in outside relationships. Bring this information back to the context of the family and suggest that this role does not appear to be working well for them any longer. Suggest that: "You deserve to be treated better. You have always deserved to be treated better. Why are you continuing the abuse the family began? What do you get and what is the price you pay for acting like a victim?"

8. Assertiveness skills training is helpful to counteract learned helplessness. Learning to take back their power, self-empowerment, is the primary means to counteract the victim role. This includes helping them be in charge of their own therapy (within your own professional boundaries, of course). This can be done by:
    a. Having the client set their own therapeutic pace, especially with respect to addressing their feelings.
    b. Having them progress on assignments.
    c. Having them set the timing of their appointment intervals.

9. Encouraging full disclosure of the abuse. Oftentimes the details of the incident hold shame, and sharing this assists them in their healing process. Work with their shame directly. Teach the client to recognize, label, and counter the shame cycle and stop the internal self-abuse (Kaufman 1980). This is a high risk time for "slips" or resuming of self-abusive behaviors. Predict and caution clients about this. Provide alternatives to old styles of coping.

10. Encouraging self-nurturing and helping them learn how to get nurturing directly from others.

11. Encouraging exploration of their feelings. (First utilize

psychometric testing to assess the ego strength of the client. If psychotic or low ego strength, do not encourage this immediately.) The basic healing process involves going back to relive the experience, reclaiming the feelings involved, and "coming out the other side" a more integrated and whole person. This can be accomplished by:
    a. Suggesting writing letters to/from the little abused child within. This part is often cut off, disenfranchised, in an effort to survive. Helping them to reconnect and own their feelings, this part of themselves.
    b. Having them visualize the incident while bringing their "adult power/helpers" to modify the result.
    c. Releasing the body's memories and tension through expressions of anger.
    d. Having them grieve their childhood losses.
    e. Encouraging drawing, writing, poems, songs — anyway to express their feelings.
    f. Writing letters to their parents (to send or not to send).
    g. Addressing how their "victim role" impacts their fear of success/failure.

12. Body work to help them reclaim their feelings and sensations. This can be accomplished by:
    a. Yoga and/or relaxation techniques
    b. Exercise
    c. Respecting and paying attention to what their bodies are telling them
    d. Self massage
    e. Professional massage
    f. Receiving nurturing/affection from others
    g. Masturbation — their right to their own sexuality

13. Later on in the therapeutic process, assisting them in looking at what (positive) they might have gotten from the abuse.
    a. In a neglectful family, this special attention is a very powerful motivator.
    b. Erotic feelings
    c. Feeling loved/cared for — Often the secret that they enjoyed part of the experience holds great shame or self-blame, as if they caused or wanted the abuse to happen.

14. If appropriate, addressing parenting skills and assessing

for possible abuse/neglect of their own children. Teaching non-shaming/non-abusive forms of discipline.

15. Even later on in the therapeutic process, after they have thoroughly processed how they were victimized, helping them look at how they were victimizers. It is helpful to place this within the context of learned behavior, within the family system, where there are only two roles (victim/victimizer) to dispel the shame/blame cycle. Look at the continuum of abuse to explore the whole range, from molestation to simple boundary violation.

16. Eventually working toward forgiveness of the abuser. The amount they continue to blame is indicative of how much they are still "hooked" into the system. Encourage decision making on what kind, if any, relationship they want to negotiate with their family. (This may or may not include family therapy to negotiate new rules.)

17. Explore spirituality (traditional or non-traditional forms). For a child who has been victimized, faith, hope and trust are oftentimes the key issues that have been damaged. Encourage development of the spiritual side of themselves.

NOTES

1. Personal correspondence.

2. Paper presented by Warren Farrell at the 6th World Congress, Washington, D.C., 1983. He reported that some family members are more likely to view their incest experience as positive. There are three groups who tend to respond in this manner: similarly-aged participants; when both participants are over age 16; and older female/younger male.

3. Minnesota Statute 609.365, Incest: whoever has sexual intercourse with another nearer of kin to him than first cousin, computed by rules of the civil law, whether of the half or the whole blood, with knowledge of the relationship, is guilty of incest and may be sentenced to imprisonment for not more than ten years.

4. These precursors are not specific to incest alone. For example, the dynamics discussed here are commonly seen in chemically dependent families as well. The authors feel that this overlap may explain in part the high correlation between chemically dependent and incestuous families.

5. Most of the symptoms listed in this assessment form, while originally developed from the author's clinical work over the past decade, are now well documented in the incest literature. For an excellent review of these studies, see Finkelhor and Browne, 1985.

ANNOTATED BIBLIOGRAPHY

1. Brady, Katherine. *Father's days.* New York: Dell Publishing Co., Inc., 1979.
   A personal account of the author's incest experience. Katherine Brady shares her feelings of shame and despair, isolation and personal responsibility resulting from her relationship with her father and the keeping of the incest secret. A clear connection is made between the sexual abuse suffered as a child with the emotional difficulties Brady struggles with as an adult. This book is cathartic for Brady, who encourages other victims to talk about their experiences and allow themselves to heal.
2. Butler, Sandra. *Conspiracy of silence – The trauma of incest.* New York: Bantam Books, 1979.
   An examination of the entire incest family in which Butler seeks to show how the secrecy surrounding incest is characteristic of abusive families and often encouraged by a society which fails to respond adequately and compassionately to the traumatic consequences of sexual abuse. The author shares several of the hundreds of interviews she held with incest victims, perpetrators and mothers. She emphasizes the vast devastation sexual abuse has on its victims, and diverse cross section of the population affected and the inadequacy and scarcity of programs set up to help them. A nationwide listing of treatment programs is provided.
3. Herbruck, Christine Comstock. *Breaking the cycle of child abuse.* Minneapolis: Winston Press, 1979.
   This book follows the recovery experiences of a small group of abusing parents and clearly demonstrates how abusive behavior is learned, passed on from one generation to the next and can, with appropriate intervention, be overcome. Through the telling of their personal stories and working through of their own childhood victimization the parents who participated in this self-help group gained insights which enabled them to connect past abuse with their present lives and find their healing in the process. Included in the book is a chapter which outlines characteristics of each of the many forms of child abuse and subsequent chapters which offer practical methods for dealing with the harmful effects of abuse.
4. Justice, Blair and Rita. *The broken taboo – Sex in the family.* New York: Human Sciences Press, 1979.
   Incestuous family dynamics are explored in this book and the authors' observations are documented with their own experiences as clinicians who have worked with hundreds of victims and offenders. Blair and Rita Justice are advocates of family recovery and claim that adequate, empathetic social and professional responses to these families will occur only when incest is desexualized and demystified. A chapter on prevention emphasizes the need for abusing parents to learn how to get their intimacy needs met, children being given the full legal right to a healthy development and the implementation of nationwide programs to help families with stress management and reduction.
5. Lewis Herman, Judith. *Father – Daughter incest.* Massachusetts: Howard University Press, 1981.
   A feminist's examination of father-daughter incest. Herman identifies and confronts an historical tendency which denies the prevalence and de-emphasizes the harmfulness of sexual activity between fathers and daughters. She challenges a tradition which defends male sexual prerogatives and emphasizes the importance of reducing male dominance, while equalizing male-female sex roles and paternal involvement in child-rearing as deterrents of sexual abuse.
6. McNaron, Toni and Morgan, Yarrow. *Voices in the night.* Minneapolis: Cleis Press, 1982.

A feminist anthology comprised of the poetry, letters, short stories and journals of 37 women who share the experience of having been sexually abused as children. McNaron and Morgan believed that there were others like themselves who found a healing in the creative expression of their incest trauma and invited women from all over the country to submit their written experiences. *Voices in the night* is the result and this collection of writing represents the voice of the incest victim, her perceptions, definitions and truths. The editors maintain that the world of the sexually abused child is a very different one from that world depicted in most literature — the body of it having been written by men. This book provides the reality of sexual abuse in an artistic form and is affirming, conscientious and intense.

7. O'Hanlon, Kacklyn. *Fair game*. New York: Dell Publishing Company, Inc., 1977.

 A fictitious account of an adolescent girl who has been sexually abused by her step-father. Centered around one isolated incident of covert abuse and the young victim's private struggle with the ensuing feelings of self-doubt, fear, shame and difficulty deciding whether or not to expose her mother's new husband. Written for adolescents, especially those who might be questioning the validity of their abuse because it was covert. Also addresses issues around protecting parents.

8. Sanford, Linda. *The silent children*. New York: McGraw-Hill Paperbacks, 1980.

 As a parents' guide to the prevention of child sexual abuse, this book offers practical suggestions to all adults interested in protecting children from victimization and enhancing their child's self-esteem. Sanford maintains that sexual abuse is the abuse of power — an adult's power over children and that children who are equipped with a sense of self-esteem, her/his own rights, as well as an understanding of sexual abuse, is less vulnerable to the sexual advances of an adult. In addition she claims that sex role stereotyping plays a part in the victimization of children by encouraging passivity in girls and discouraging boys from trusting their feelings. The book concludes with a chapter which provides parents with a method of discussing sexual abuse with their children in a non-threatening way. Also includes suggestions for educating children with special needs.

9. Schultz, Leroy G. *The sexual victimology of youth*. Charles G. Thomas, 1980.

 This book offers a composite of important information on sexual child abuse. Shultz records medical models drawn from emergency room cases and gynecological cases, illustrating various modes, and consequences of sexual abuse of children. Recognition of rape, incest, child molestation and other sexual trauma of children are drawn out and exposed in this book. It includes shocking statistics on the sexual victimology of people under the age of 15 years.

10. Walker, Alice. *The color purple*. Harcourt Brace Jovanovich, 1982.

 A fictitious but truly powerful novel about incest and the impact it has on a child growing up with very little support. The dialogue imparts great emotional content into the story line and gives the reader insight into the mental and emotional workings of an incest victim.

ADDITIONAL READINGS

1. Hamner, Signe. *Daughters and mothers/Mothers and daughters*. Signet Books, 1976.

 This book is included because it indicates how boundaries between mothers and daughters impact emotional health. Hamner examines the relationship between mothers and daughters and how dependency conflicts can follow throughout both women's lives. She reveals the fear of separation and the anger of "double messages" given by the mother to her daughter. It is good on boundary issues, good for women looking at their relationships to their own mothers/to their own daughters or both.

2. Kaufman, Gershen. *Shame – The power of caring.* Shenkman Publishing Co., Inc., 1980.

One of the better sources of information regarding shame and how to recover from its impact. The author gives concise examples of shame, shame-based identities, and the therapeutic process whereby one can begin the healing process.

3. Kaplan, Louise. *Oneness and separateness: From infant to individual.* Simon and Schuster, 1978.

This is an excellent book on boundary development in that it explores the relationship between the primary care giver and child from birth to three years of age. It describes the developmental process of the child and its typical behaviors at each stage. In addition, it explores the typical and atypical responses of the parent in the early phase and its impact on the mental health of the child. The book goes into depth about the separation and individuation process that is so vital to developing boundaries.

4. Kerr, Carmen. *Sex for women.* New York: Grove Press, Inc., 1977.

Designed as a guidebook for women who want to rediscover, enhance and enjoy their sexuality, Kerr defines sexuality as a "personal power" often dormant in women who have internalized the rigid rules, roles and expectations of our sexist society. Feminist insight is applied to transactional analysis in an effort to help women identify and rid themselves of those inherited or imposed attitudes and behaviors which impair sexual enjoyment. The last chapters of the book provide a program for personal sexual development and emphasize the need for women to discover value and assume responsibility for their own sexual needs.

5. Kopp, Sheldon. *Mirror, mask and shadow.* Bantam Books, 1980.

Kopp, through personal experiences and his recordings of client experiences, explains the trials and tribulations of self-discovery and acceptance. He examines the reasons why we wear a mask to maintain a social self-image that feels acceptable to us, but not necessarily to other people. He then goes on to explain how we see ourselves through others people in society, our "mirrors." Finally, after revealing his own shadow, Kopp describes fear of this shadow, but he also exposes the relevation that comes with discovering and then accepting our true selves. This book provides another view of shame.

REFERENCES

Bible. Genesis 19:26, 19:30-36 See also: Geiser, R. *Hidden victims.* Boston: Beacon Press, 1979.

Benward, J. and Densen-Gerber, J. Incest as a causative factor in antisocial behavior: An exploratory study. *Contemporary Drug Problems,* 4: 323-340, 1975.

Browning, D. H. & Boatman, B. Incest: Children at risk. *American Journal of Psychiatry,* 134: 69-72, 1977.

Butler, S. *Conspiracy of silence.* California: New Glide Publications, 1978.

Cavallin, H. Incestuous fathers: A clinical report. *American Journal of Psychiatry, 134*: 1132-1138, 1966.

Coleman, E. Family intimacy and chemical abuse: The connection. *Journal of Psychoactive Drugs, 14,* 1982, pp. 153-158.

Coleman, E. & Colgan, P. Boundary inadequacy in chemically dependent families. *Journal of Psychoactive Drugs*, 1986.
Finkelhor, David, PhD and Brown, Angela, PhD. The traumatic impact of child sexual abuse: A conceptualization. *American Journal of Orthopsychiatry*, 1985, 55, 530.
Hammer, S. *Daughters and mothers: Mothers and daughters*. New York: Signet, 1976.
Hammond, D. C., Jorgenson, G. Q., and Ridgeway, D. M. "Sexual Adjustment of the Female Alcoholic." Unpublished manuscript. Salt Lake City Alcohol and Drug Abuse Clinic, University of Utah, 1979.
Hayek, M. A. "Recovering Alcoholic Women With and Without Incest Experience: A Comparative Study." Unpublished doctoral dissertation, Reed University, 1980.
Kaufman, G. *Shame-The power of caring*. Cambridge, MA: Schenkman Publishing Co., Inc., 1980.
Kaplan, L. J. *Oneness and separateness: From infant to individual*. New York: Simon and Schuster, 1978.
Kopp, S. *Mirror, mask and shadow*. New York: Macmillan Publishing Company, Inc., 1980.
Miller, A. *Prisoners of Childhood*. Basic Books, Inc., 1981. English Translation.
Rosenfeld, A. A., Nadelson, C. C., Krieger, M. & Blackman, J. H. Incest and sexual abuse of children. *Journal of Child Psychiatry*, 1977, *16*, 327-339.
Sterne, M., Schaefer, S. and Evans, S. Women's Sexuality and alcoholism. In P. Golding (Ed.) *Alcoholism: Analysis of a world-wide problem*. Lancaster, England: MTP Press Limited-International Medical Publishers, 1983.
Summit, R., Kryso, J. Sexual abuse of children: A clinical spectrum. *American Journal of Orthopsychiatry*, 1978, *48*, 237-251.
Virkkunen, M. Incest offenses and alcoholism. *Medical Science and the Law, 14*: 124-128, 1974.
Weber, E. Incest begins at home. *MS*. 5 (2 bound) (10 unbound): 64-67 + 105, 1977.
Weinberg, S. K. *Incest Behavior*. New Jersey: The Citadel Press, 1976.
Wilsnack, S. Femininity by the bottle. *Psychology Today*. 6(1): 39-43, 1973.

Identifying the Male Chemically Dependent Sex Offender and a Description of Treatment Methods

Margretta Dwyer, RSM, MA

Achieving intimacy in relationships is usually a problem for chemically dependent persons. Many believe that when chemical dependency is addressed all other problems will be alleviated. Attending Alcoholics Anonymous meetings and announcing frequently that "I am a recovering alcoholic" are often seen as the "magic" that will keep people chemically free and help them build intimate relationships. Indeed, this is partially true. However, if some problems such as sex offending behaviors are not addressed during chemical dependency treatment, then rehabilitation is jeopardized and further growth is arrested.

The folklore of AA appears to be: "The AA goal is abstinence above and beyond anything else, including . . . family relationships. Don't drink, go to meetings, and pray, in that order. You cannot handle problems if you drink. If you don't drink they may get better" (Holland, 1985). The author's clinical experience is that sexual misconduct problems do not get better solely by abstinence from alcohol or involvement in Alcoholics Anonymous. Sexual problems will remain and may even get worse. Sex offenders may complete a second or third chemical dependency treatment, attend Alcoholics Anonymous meetings several times

---

Margretta Dwyer is the Coordinator of the Sex Offender Treatment Program at the Program in Human Sexuality, Department of Family Practice and Community Health, Medical School, University of Minnesota, 2630 University Avenue, S.E., Minneapolis, MN 55414.

The author wishes to acknowledge the help of Lianne Smith in editing and preparing this manuscript.

© 1987 by The Haworth Press, Inc. All rights reserved.

a week and "keep the cork in the bottle" for a time, but later begin drinking again due to underlying sexual problems.

There are numerous reasons why someone may return again and again for chemical dependency treatment. Only one of these issues will be addressed; that is, the sex offender who has been able to maintain the secrecy of his sexual offenses throughout his chemical dependency treatment. The author's experience is that treating chemical dependency without treating the sex offending problem leads a person back to drinking and consequentially back into another chemical dependency treatment program.

PATTERNS OF A SEX OFFENDER

Before discussing how sex offenders avoid sexual issues during chemical dependency treatment, the patterns of a sex offender must be examined. Following are fourteen patterns frequently found in a sex offender (Dwyer, Amberson & Seabloom, 1985).

1. A tremendous disdain for sex offenders exists among the offender population, therefore, the defense mechanism of denial must operate constantly in the sex offender's system in order to avoid thinking of himself as one of these "horrible" people.
2. Offenders have a very poor or nonexistent relationship with their fathers, and they often were ignored by their fathers throughout early development, thereby missing any nurturing touch from a male.
3. Offenders often had overprotective mothers and have later in their lives sought out overprotective partners who become primary enablers in their lives. Both the men and their partners contribute to this unhealthy interaction.
4. Offenders have usually experienced an early sexual trauma that contributes to their aberrant behavior. They develop their acting-out behavior as a way to "triumph over this trauma" (Stoller, 1975), and it becomes part of their sexual pattern.
5. Approximately 56% (this is thought to be underestimated) of these men reported they were sexually abused as children.

6. Obsessive moral religious codes are used by these men to enable them to violate socially acceptable norms, yet keep them from psychologically normal activities (e.g., masturbation).
7. Most offenders are immature in either social or sexual skills, or both.
8. Offenders generally exhibit low self-esteem and high self-criticism.
9. Sexuality is seen as something separate and outside of themselves.
10. Offenders see their behavior as though it were someone else acting, enabling them to dissociate themselves in yet another way from who they are.
11. Offenders are generally passive and are unable to make forceful decisions. This passivity further encourages the overprotective mother and/or spouse to make the decisions.
12. There is an inability to appropriately express anger. Tremendous amounts of repressed anger exist within their personalities, yet these men have great feelings of intimidation when with other adult males or females.
13. Repression is a defense mechanism that is consistently used by the offender for his fantasy life and for sexuality in general. The offender thinks that repressing sexual thoughts will prevent his acting out.
14. Offenders use manipulation as a tool to protect the dual lifestyle they must lead. An offender might operate as an upstanding businessman in the community and yet in his private life, be sexual with children or expose himself, etc.

Given these characteristics, a major personality revision is required. However, with a proper treatment plan, the prognosis is good.

DEMOGRAPHICS

Data for this paper is based on the male sex offender population at the University of Minnesota's Program in Human Sexuality. The age range is between 18 and 72 with the mean age being 35. Ninety percent are white, 55.7% are married, 38.6% have only one sexual partner, and 73% have been married once. Fourteen percent attended a trade school, 20% have had some college, and 29% are college graduates. They are a mixture of rural and urban persons, and 74.3% claim a current affiliation with a religion.

PERCENTAGE WHO ARE CHEMICALLY DEPENDENT

Many believe that a majority—or that all—sex offenders are chemically dependent. Our experience does not support this view. The majority of sex offenders do not have a problem with alcohol or other drugs. Approximately 33% of 140 sex offenders studied at our clinic did have a diagnosis of chemical dependency, and a majority of these were incest fathers. Our data indicates that approximately 90-95% of incest fathers were either alcoholic or were periodically abusing alcohol at the time of the offenses. From our clinical experience, generally other pedophiles do not have this problem.

TREATMENT ISSUES

Sex offenders mainly use the defense mechanisms of repression, manipulation, and denial which enables them to keep their secret. Using these defense mechanisms, they can often cleverly complete chemical dependency treatment and never admit to improper sexual behavior. When offending sexual behaviors (or issues of sexuality in general) are not explored, it is the author's clinical experience that the patient will recirculate through another chemical dependency treatment program. All of our alcoholic patients who did not mention their sexual problems during their first chemical dependency treatment believe this was the reason necessitating a second chemical dependency treatment. The haunting experience of being a pedophile (someone who is sexually aroused by children), a voyeur, an exhibitionist, an incest perpetrator, or other offender is so frightening and upsetting to the recovering chemical dependency individual that he begins to drink again in an attempt to not reoffend by "erasing" the arousing thoughts.

If issues of sexuality are not addressed by the professional, the patient will find it difficult to bring up this topic on his own initiative. Admitting to being a sex offender is frightening; therefore, having the chemical dependency professional ask some leading questions in the area of sexuality gives a patient the opportunity to confide that he or she has a sexual problem or may have committed sexual offenses. The chemical dependency professional should be aware that most will say "it only happened one time" or "I only exposed one time" or "I was a voyeur one time." This claim to having "only done it once" often occurs in the initial interaction between patient and therapist. Because of the tendency of the offender to conceal sex offenses, counselors should take an extensive sexual history over a period of several sessions. The fact that so many of our chemically dependent sex offenders have been through three or four chemical dependency treatments before sexual issues are addressed is a tremendous oversight in the mental health system.

WHICH COMES FIRST

In treating sex offenders, chemical dependency treatment must come first. Much to their credit, no sex offender treatment program this author knows of will consider a person for sex offender treatment until the issue of chemical dependency has been resolved. The reasons for this are obvious. First, treatment cannot be effective while their minds and senses are sedated with drugs. Second, active alcoholism will most likely continue to perpetuate the sex offending behavior. Finally, typical sex offender treatment programs are lengthy—approximately two years, some longer. During this time a person must be chemically free in order to *fully* participate in the therapeutic process.

ASSESSMENT

At the University of Minnesota, Program in Human Sexuality there are group therapy sessions, family, family of origin, and individual therapy sessions. Therapy sessions with victims are conducted when appropriate. The patient and partner are also required to attend a two-day educational "Sexual Attitude Reassessment Seminar." Since most sexual offenders have legal problems, meetings with probation officers are held quarterly. Throughout the intake and therapy process, the patient is subjected to numerous questionnaires, psychological tests, and laboratory tests. To engage in this much therapy and to regularly attend sessions and profit from them, the patient must not be abusing chemicals. By taking a complete sex history and asking blunt questions regarding exhibitionism, voyeurism, pedophilia, incest, or other paraphilias, the professional will obtain important therapeutic information. Chemical dependency programs either need to have people who are trained in sex therapy to make these assessments, or they need to work in conjunction with a clinic that offers sexual problem assessments.

Once sex offending behavior is diagnosed and the patient has completed chemical dependency treatment, the chemical dependency professional can enable the patient to look for an appropriate sex offender treatment program. When looking for an appropriate sex offender treatment, the need for inpatient treatment or outpatient treatment must clearly be assessed. Some offenders need more controls put on them at the beginning of treatment than others, and consequently they may be successful only in an inpatient treatment program. However, the sex offender treatment program itself will be able to determine whether inpatient or outpatient treatment is needed. If there is any doubt about inpatient treatment being needed most therapists take the conservative side and use an inpatient program. Research indicates, and our experience shows, that most sex offenders can be treated in an outpatient sex offenders program.

KEY ELEMENTS OF A TREATMENT PROGRAM

Group therapy is considered to be a key tool in treating offenders and absolutely essential for their progress (Dwyer, Amberson & Seabloom, 1985). Truax (1970), known for his work in group therapy, states that it is extremely important for sex offenders to be in a group of people with similar problems, needs, and common experiences. The group experience enables the participants to penetrate the defense mechanisms of rationalization, isolation, and denial. Individual therapy encourages the hiding of information, lessens the ability to share difficult thoughts and feelings, and promotes the keeping of secrets which feeds into the defense mechanism of repression and denial. This cycle can trap the offender into obsessing more about his secrets (Dwyer, Amberson & Seabloom, 1985). Therefore, group psychotherapy for sex offenders has been encouraged by many (Turner, 1961; Rosen, 1964; Mathis & Collin, 1970). It is widely accepted that this is the only method that is successful with the manipulative sex offending personality.

As far back as 1926, research indicated that treatment for the sex offender should be compulsory (Staeagilin, 1926; Mathis & Collin, 1970). Sex offender treatment is difficult and long; the offender is expanding his personality, learning new behaviors, and searching all the way back to his early developmental years for clues about who he is. This difficult work leads many offenders to want to quit in the middle of therapy. But if therapy is compulsory, they know they must come back next week to continue on this long voyage. This author's experience is that volunteers in the sex offender treatment program tend not to be successful and tend to leave treatment too early.

Furthermore, it has been shown that a male and female therapist should be used in the group (Mathis & Collin, 1970). Male and female therapists are role models in the group. For many of the men it is the first time they have had to interact with a female in appropriate, assertive ways and confront them when they are displeased. Also, it is the first time many of the offenders have interacted in a very personal way with a female without being sexual. The male therapist serves as a model for teaching the men feelings, caring about their bodies, and being affectionate. Through both the male and female therapists, these men learn appropriate touch and come to understand that affection toward males and affection toward females needn't have sexual overtures. If only male therapists are used, a large component of learning about women will be missing from the therapy. A female co-therapist is essential in group therapy in order to model appropriate female behavior and to help counteract the negative beliefs and stereotypes that these men have about women (Schwartz & Masters, 1983).

Research on the effectiveness of aversion therapy indicates that the use of noxious stimuli, painful electrical stimulation, or any form of aversion therapy, does not produce long-term benefits (Bancroft, 1969).

In analyzing earlier-described patterns of the offender, it is important that a treatment program be structured in a way that changes these patterns or eliminates them altogether. Therefore, it is essential that many modalities of therapy be incorporated into a competent treatment program.

TREATMENT MODALITIES

In an appropriate treatment program, several treatment modalities should be present. (Figure 1 and Figure 2 describe a comprehensive treatment program.)

Psychodynamic Therapy

It is important to pierce through the unconscious motives that the offender may have for his behavior. The patient analyzes himself and his early childhood learning, family of origin lifestyles, and critical developmental periods. In this mode he analyzes the traumatic event that may have contributed to the development of his specific offending behavior, although he may have no understanding of its importance, or even remember the event when first starting therapy (Stoller, 1975).

Social Skills Training

Development of social skills should be incorporated into a good treatment program. During this time the client can learn the basic skills of relating to others, thereby filling in long-standing deficits regarding assertiveness and social interaction. This modality can be enhanced with the use of television monitors, role-playing, and using the group's help for self-analysis (Dwyer, Amberson & Seabloom, 1985). Once again, the need for group therapy is essential in teaching a variety of verbal and non-verbal behaviors (Abel, Blanchard & Becker, 1977; Eisler, Miller & Hersen, 1973).

Behavior Modification Therapy

Since the offender has behavioral excesses or deficits (Eisler, Miller & Hersen, 1973), measurable homework assignments involving behavior modification must be given both in group and in family therapy sessions. These behaviors are practiced during the ensuing weeks and checked on in group and family therapy. Us-

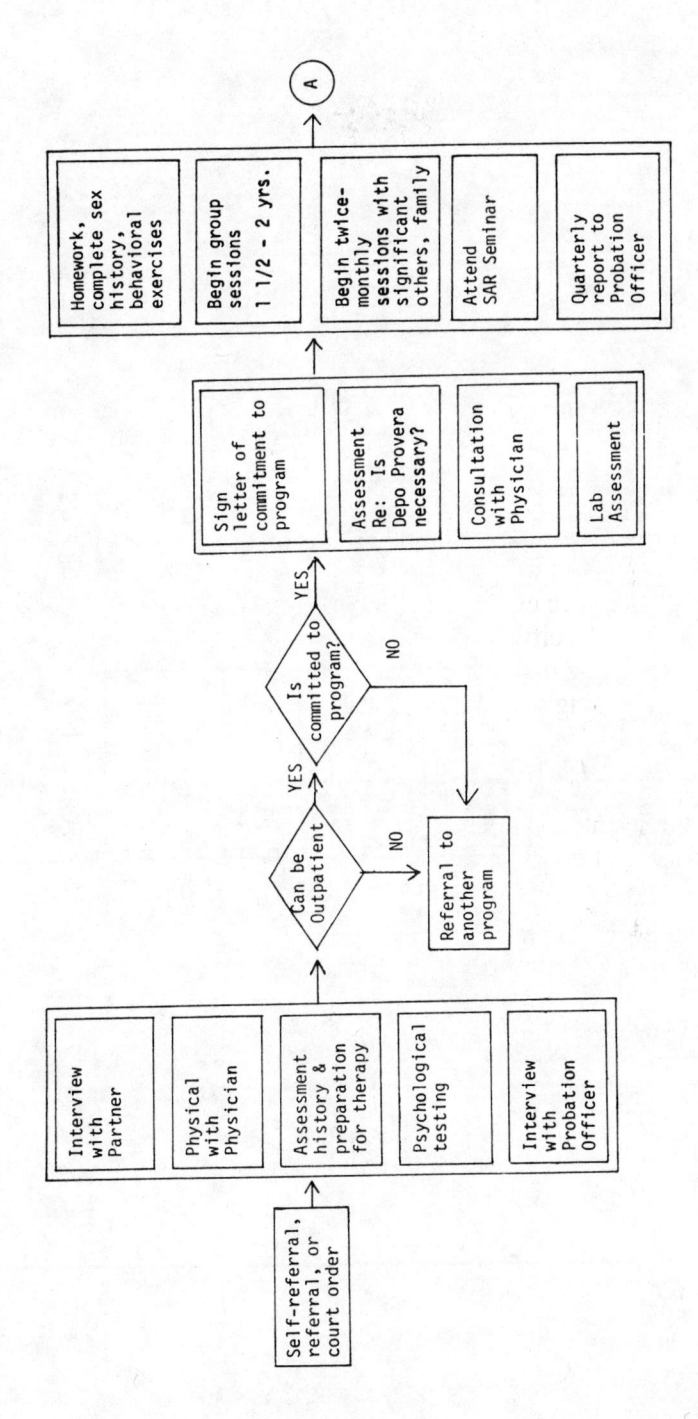

Figure 1. Sex Offender Program Flow Chart Part 1.

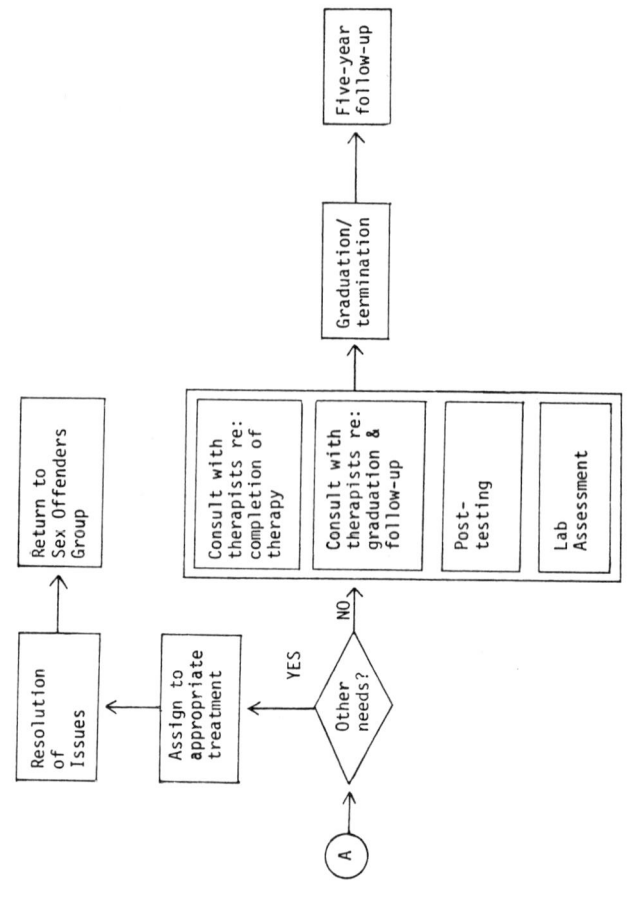

Figure 2. Sex Offender Program Flow Chart Part 2.

ing reciprocal inhibition to extinguish a neurotic response to a given stimulus and thereby to obtain a new response is a useful form of therapy that should be incorporated into behavioral treatment (Wolpe, 1958). Thoughtstopping, relaxation exercises, ways to lessen anxiety, and other such behaviors can be taught. It is essential that these specific tasks assigned are followed up on in the group setting (Barlow & Abel, 1976).

Learning to touch is very difficult for offenders, and in the past touch has often been associated with rough, aggressive touch or sexual offending touch. Appropriate touching also must be taught (Abel, 1976; Able, Blanchard & Becker, 1977).

In all areas of behavior modification reinforcement — not punishment — should be consistently used. The offender should be taught to manage stress without retreating into fantasy (Schwartz & Masters, 1973).

Cognitive Therapy

Changing the patient's maladaptive cognitions is an essential part of the therapy in order for the patient to acquire new behaviors. Group members help a patient scrutinize the validity of his assumptions and examine whether his experiences are realistic or whether he needs to make some cognitive changes.

Structural and Strategic Family Therapy

Poor relationships within the family are a reoccurring theme in the sex offender population. It is essential that family therapy sessions be scheduled at least two to four times a month. The approaches of a variety of family therapists can be used including those of Haley, Minunchin, Whitaker, and Erickson, to name a few. It is often necessary to include the sex offender's family of origin as well as his present nuclear family.

Hormonal/Physiological Treatment

A good sex offender treatment program will incorporate hormonal treatment if it is needed. This therapy should be available to a patient even though it is seldom used in outpatient programs. Much research needs to be done yet to explore fully the advantages or disadvantages of drug therapy. However, to enable some men to relax, and decrease their sexual desires, fantasies, and acting-out behavior, it may be necessary to administer the drug Depo-Provera, an anti-androgenic agent. This drug is commonly administered for a short period of time, six months at most. This drug is not approved by the F.D.A. and, therefore, can be offered to the patient only with his consent and his full knowledge of its lack of F.D.A. approval and possible side effects. This drug is titrated according to an individual's body weight. It usually takes approximately a month before the effects are felt or noticed.

CONCLUSION

Treating only a chemical abuse problem will not alleviate a sexual problem. This is particularly true of psychosexual disorders that include sex offending behaviors. The greatest issue surrounding many sex offenders therefore, is not alcohol but rather multiple personality and family problems together; with a lack of appropriate social skills and dysfunctional psychosexual development. When these problems are treated, stress decreases and psychosexual functioning and interpersonal functioning improves and the patient then has a greater chance of recovering from chemical dependency.

REFERENCES

Abel, G. G. (1976) Assessment of sexual deviation in the male. In M. Hershen & A. S. Bellack, (Eds.), *Behavioral assessment: A practice handbook* (pp. 437-457). New York: Pergamon Press.
Abel, G. G., Becker, J. & Cunningham-Rathner, J. (1984). Complications, consent, and cognitions in sex between children and adults. *International Journal of Law & Psychiatry,* 7, 89-103.
Abel, G. G., Blanchard, E. B. & Becker, J. V. (1977). An integrated treatment program for rapists. In R. T. Rada (Ed.), *Clinical aspects of the rapist* (pp. 161-213). Grune & Stratton.
Bancroft, J. (1969). Aversion therapy of homosexuality: A pilot study of ten cases. *British Journal of Psychiatry,* 115, 1417-1431.
Barlow, D. H., & Abel, G. G. (1976). Sexual deviation. In A. Kandin, M. Mahoney, & E. Craighead (Eds.) *Behavior Modification: Principles, issues, and applications* (pp. 341-360). Boston: Houghton Mifflin.
Dwyer, S. M., Amberson, I. J. & Seabloom, W. (1985). A theoretical base for a sex offender treatment program. Manuscript submitted for publication.

Eisler, R. N., Miller, P. M., & Hersen, M. (1973). Components of assertive behavior. *Journal of Clinical Psychology, 29*, 295-299.
Holland, V. J. (1985). The invisible problem. *Family Therapy Networker, 9*(6), 15.
Schwartz, M. F. & Masters, D. H. (1983, Spring). Conceptual factors in the treatment of paraphilias: A preliminary report. *Journal of Sex and Marital Therapy*.
Stahelin, J. E. (1926). Untersuchungen an 70 Exhibtionisten. *Zschr. f.d. ges. Neur. u. Psychiatrie*. Germany.
Stoller, R. J., (1975). *Perversion: The erotic form of hatred*. New York: Pantheon Books.
Wolpe, J. (1958). *Therapy by reciprocal inhibition*. London: Oxford University Press.

Sexual Compulsivity: Definition, Etiology, and Treatment Considerations

Eli Coleman, PhD

SUMMARY. While no consensus on the definition or method of assessing sexual compulsivity exists, there is a growing realization that certain sexual behavior patterns could become the agent for compulsive disorders. This paper reviews the controversy over definition and conceptualization and offers a hypothesized definition of sexual compulsivity, etiology and treatment methodology. One high risk group for developing sexually compulsive behavior patterns is chemically dependent individuals and their family members. The reasons for this higher incidence rate among this group are explained and professionals are urged to look for symptoms of sexual compulsivity and look for treatment opportunities as simply treating the chemical dependence or co-dependence will rarely alter this symptomology.

Sex, like a quick "fix," can be a coping mechanism or an escape similar to alcohol or drugs. Sex can serve as an anesthetic to psychological pain. It can be a way of feeling good quickly. It can mask low self-esteem and lack of intimacy in the person's life, even seem to create a false sense of intimacy. Sex, in short, can distract the individual from the painful realities of life. When sex is used to bypass the development of self-esteem and intimacy in relationships, the individual remains frozen in insecurity

---

Dr. Coleman is the Associate Director and Associate Professor at the Program in Human Sexuality, Department of Family Practice and Community Health, Medical School, University of Minnesota, 2630 University Ave. S.E., Minneapolis, MN 55414.
Reprint requests may be obtained by contacting the author at the address listed above.
The author would like to acknowledge the assistance of Orlo Otteson in preparing the manuscript.

© 1987 by The Haworth Press, Inc. All rights reserved.

and never develops a positive and integrated identity. More pain results and the need continues to numb the pain, to search for instant solutions, to find the high to distract oneself from oneself. When the individual compulsively looks to sex to solve these problems, or to become medicated against them, the preoccupation with sex serves not only as a barrier to intimacy but also eventually destroys what intimacy the individual has been able to enjoy in life.

Everyone must experience sexuality in some way to survive. Children and older people who do not receive touch will fail to thrive and ultimately die. In this sense sex is a necessity of life, just as air, food, and warmth. However, the sexually compulsive individual does not simply depend on sex to survive and satisfy his or her body's need. He or she compulsively seeks out sexual activity in order to cope with, to forget about, to escape from, to anesthetize the pain of his or her life. Sex initially accomplishes those goals but inevitably loses its effectiveness and produces more pain, because of the negative effects caused by the compulsive drive. The individual, searches to triumph over the traumas of his or her life, ends up further traumatized. It is a pathetic, frustrated, hopeless search. Without recognition of the problem and redirection, the individual continues to suffer.

DEFINITION

There is no consensus on the definition or method of assessing sexual compulsivity (Coleman, 1986). Yet, there has been a growing realization that sexual behaviors could become the agent for compulsive disorders. No consensus exists whether these behavior patterns could be described as psychosexual, obsessive-compulsive personality, impulse, or addictive disorders. How to describe these behavior patterns is still under debate and discussion. What is clear is that a number of people are concerned about the excesses, the lack of control, the amount of preoccupation, and the disruption of their lives as a result of their pattern of expression of sexual behavior. For now, this author utilizes some of the dynamics of other compulsive or addictive behaviors as criteria for sexual compulsivity. A person who is sexually compulsive is obsessively preoccupied with certain patterns of sexual behavior and as a result of this preoccupation, experiences negative consequences following engaging in this behavior. Yet, in spite of the negative consequences, the individual experiences great difficulty and many frustrated attempts to change his or her behavior. Individuals become preoccupied with sexual behavior such as pornography, prostitution, masturbation, sexual intercourse, affairs, anonymous sexual encounters, and certain fetishistic behaviors. Some typical consequences of engaging in these behaviors in compulsive patterns are arrest, loss of job, relationships and self-esteem, and illness or physical injury.

Any sexual behavior can become compulsive. This understanding of sexual compulsivity avoids making value judgments about any type of sexual behavior (e.g., prostitution, sadomasochism, cross-dressing, affairs, anonymous sex). These behaviors could be healthy expressions of sexuality as well as potentially abusive or compulsive. The pattern of the behavior, the motivation and the result determine whether a behavior is a healthy use of the behavior, abusive, or compulsive. Sexual intercourse between a married couple could become a compulsive behavior. For example, a man who becomes preoccupied with sexual intercourse with his wife and insists on sexual intercourse three times a day could be considered sexually compulsive. Trying other types of sexual activity with his wife or varying this schedule are simply frustrating. He must have this activity or he becomes very agitated, anxious or depressed. To avoid these uncomfortable feelings, he will go to great lengths to ensure he gets his "fix." He might spend hours convincing his wife to have sexual intercourse with him or he may resort to violence.

Another example could be the married man who spends hours a day "cruising" streets looking for prostitutes. The moment he wakes up in the morning, he is thinking about the type of woman he wants to pick up that day. As he says goodbye to his wife in the morning, he fantasizes what she would be like if she were a prostitute. He goes to work and is frustrated because his work must be done and he cannot go directly to find a prostitute. He is extremely relieved at lunch time when he has a chance to cruise the streets. He finds someone. He has sex with her in a hotel room, then finds himself looking for another on his way back to work.

Another example could be the single woman who has repeated anonymous sexual encounters. Her entire life revolves around finding the next man. She begins the day by imagining what clothes will be the most alluring. On the bus to work, she cruises most of the men, even the ones she doesn't find particularly attractive. Walking down the aisle to get off the bus, she brushes her buttocks on men she passes. At work, she flirts with the security guard. She becomes so preoccupied with the elevator operator that she forgets to get off on her floor. She gives him her phone number and insists he call her that night. At lunch, she heads to one of the singles lunch places. Within minutes, she begins a conversation with a fairly attractive man and they leave to go to his apartment. She calls work and tells them she has become ill and won't be back to work that afternoon. The story continues . . .

TREATMENT APPROACHES

As a result of a greater recognition of this problem, there has been a growing number of self-help and professional treatment programs. These treatment approaches have spawned books, articles, television programs, and lively discussions among sexual scientists and professionals in the addiction field addressing these concerns.

There has been a rather overwhelming increase in the number of self-help groups designed to help people who are concerned about their lack of control and destructive patterns of sex behavior. These groups have been designed to help participants to gain control over these patterns of behavior. Many of the methods of these groups have been borrowed from the 12 steps and traditions of Alcoholics Anonymous (AA). In the 12 Steps of AA, members are asked to take a first step and acknowledge that they are powerless over alcohol and that their lives have become unmanageable. In Sex Addicts Anonymous (SAA), for example, this first step is simply changed to, "We admitted we were powerless over our sexual addiction — that our lives had become unmanageable." The remainder of the 12 Steps of AA remain the same. This group, as well as others, borrows heavily from the AA and Alanon literature and has been found so helpful to many alcoholics and people around them. As the literature for Sex Addicts Anonymous states,

> Sex Addicts Anonymous (SAA) is a fellowship of men and women who are committed to a program of spiritual recovery from a life that invited compulsive, uncontrollable, and harmful sexual practices.
>
> It is not aligned with any religion, sect or denomination. It is not affiliated with any program or organization, and neither accepts or receives any financial support aside from the voluntary contributions of its members. We carry our message of hope to other sex addicts who seek our help.
>
> *Twin Cities SAA*
> *P.O. Box 3038*
> *Minneapolis, Minnesota 55403*

There are numerous other self-help organizations with little or no connection to each other. These are grass-roots organizations and they often have little contact with one another. Furthermore, while usually adhering to an addiction model for understanding the sexual behavior of their members, they often differ significantly in philosophy and method. It should not be assumed that one group operates like another—even in the same organization and city. Some of the names of these organizations have been called, "Sex Addicts Anonymous," "Sexaholics Anonymous," "Sex and Love Anonymous," and "Sex Abusers Anonymous."

Various professional treatment programs have also significantly increased in number. These treatment programs are sometimes inpatient or outpatient facilities and they often differ significantly in terms of treatment philosophy and method. Some programs utilize psychoanalytic, social-learning, family systems, cognitive, behavioral, and/or biological treatments. Some programs utilize an addiction model borrowed from the methods to treat alcoholics, while others use models of treating obsessive-compulsive or impulse control disorders. Some utilize hormonal therapy—in particular the use of depo-provera (an anti-androgenic agent). Some treatment programs distinguish between individuals who are "compulsive" or "addictive" sex offenders (e.g., rapists, exhibitionists, incest perpetrators, etc.) and those with less social or criminal offenses with the same "compulsive" or "addictive" characteristics such as (masturbation, multiple sexual partners, etc.). All combinations are possible and so each program is usually different and unique to some degree. There is no consensus at present or much research demonstrating treatment effectiveness.

THE DEBATE OVER TERMINOLOGY

There has been quite a debate regarding terminology which reflects some of the philosophical differences in psychological theory underlying the understanding of these patterns of behaviors (Coleman, 1986; Carnes, 1986). "Sexual Addiction" has received the most discussion as it was one of the first of the new generation of terminology and popularized by the printing of Patrick Carnes', PhD, book entitled, "The Sexual Addiction," now retitled, "Out of the Shadows: Understanding the Sexual Addict" (1983). John Money, PhD (1985), at Johns Hopkins Hospital and School of Medicine, has indicated that it is the object of erotic passion (or the person) to which someone becomes addicted. In the paraphilias, the love partner becomes replaced, in part or in toto, by some intrusion. A fetish, for example, a shoe fetish, insists on being included in the imagery of erotic arousal. A fetishist is addicted to his fetish.

Essentially, the criticism and the danger of describing sex as an addiction is that it presupposes that the individual is addicted to all forms of sexual behavior rather than a specific sexual object or set of sexual behaviors. And following the addiction model, suggests abstinence as a treatment goal.

Others have viewed these patterns of behavior as sexual compulsions (Quadland, 1985a, 1985b). Dr. David Barlow (1985) has described these as obsessive-compulsive disorders. Others, such as Dr. Andrew Mattison at the Clinical Institute of Human Relationships in San Diego have preferred a non-diagnostic labeling of these behaviors and to simply describe them as "Problems of Sexual Control."

As indicated earlier, what this pattern of behavior is called is indicative of a theoretical orientation. While sexual scientists debate this question, the author's clients seem to be most comfortable with either describing their problems as compulsions or addictions. Nevertheless, the importance of the debate over terminology must continue to achieve greater understanding and treatment methodology and success.

It should be noted that many concerns and arguments have been made against any such conceptualization of sex as a potential agent for a compulsive or addictive behavior (e.g., Cushman, 1985; Sharon, 1985; Taylor, 1985; Wedin, 1985a, 1985b; and Levine, 1985).

Consequently, this author has tried to caution his clients and other professionals about the problems of the labelling process and admit our lack of knowledge regarding these problems. However, this author is willing to treat people who are in psychological distress because they perceive their sex behavior as having the elements of preoccupation, lack of control and destructiveness to their well-being or their lives. There is also a recognition that sexual behavior should be viewed on a continuum (see Figure 1); for every sexual behavior has its healthy aspects and its potential for abuse or compulsion. (At this point, I prefer the term abusive behavior patterns or compulsivity because there seems to be more uncertainty and potential harm for the use of the term addiction. If I am to use the term addiction, I prefer to use terminology such as "like an addiction," or "addiction-like.")

HEALTHY	ABUSIVE	COMPULSIVE
Self-enhancing	Self-limiting	Self-limiting
Productive	Unproductive	Unproductive
Enjoyable	Unenjoyable	Unenjoyable
Within value system	Outside Value System	Outside Value System
		Self Destructive
		Other-destructive
		Preoccupation
		Obsessive
		Negative Consequences
FEELINGS	FEELINGS	FEELINGS
Satisfaction	Temporary "Fix"	Dissatisfaction
Pleasure	Discomfort	Discomfort
Fulfillment	Emptiness	Emptiness
	Guilt	Guilt
		Shame
		Hopeless
		Desparate
		Suicidal

Figure 1. Continuum of Sexual Compulsivity

ETIOLOGY

The etiology of this still ill-defined set of behaviors is obviously obscure. But in a scientific fashion, I have my own hypotheses based upon existing theoretical notions of compulsivity and addictions and descriptive data based upon my own clinical sample. In my clinical experience, some type of historical family intimacy dysfunction or abuse can be found (see Figure 2). In response to this trauma, the client begins to develop feelings of shame (Coleman, 1986). Somehow, they perceive that they were the cause of the abuse—whether it was neglect, physical, psychological, sexual or emotional abuse. They develop feelings of unworthiness and a feeling that somehow their personality is inherently defective (see Gershwin Kaufman, 1980, for a better description of this process). This feeling of shame obviously results in low self-esteem and an interruption in normal, healthy interpersonal functioning—leaving the person feeling lonely. All of these events and feelings cause psychological pain for the client. And, in order to alleviate this pain, the client begins to search for a "fix," or an agent which has analgesic qualities to it. For some, this agent is alcohol. For others, it could be drugs,

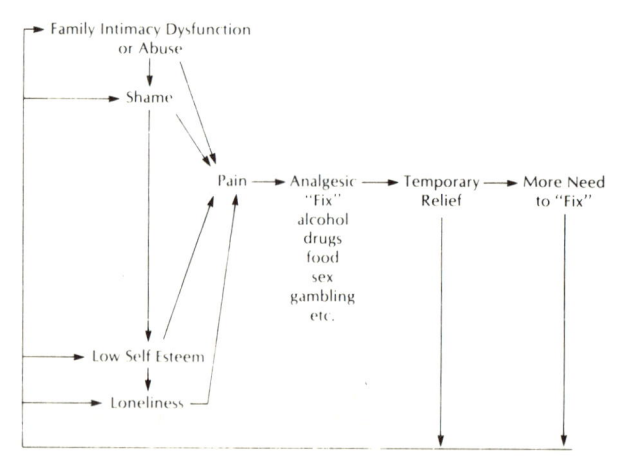

FIGURE 2. Development of compulsive behavior patterns.

certain sexual behaviors, particular foods, working patterns, gambling behaviors, etc. All seem to cause physical and psychological changes which alleviate the pain and provide a temporary relief. This respite from the psychological pain wears off and the shame, low self-esteem and loneliness return. Thus, there is the increased need to return to the temporarily relieving "fix." The behavior becomes repetitious and forms a vicious cycle which simply feeds a greater need to engage in the behavior for its analgesic qualities. Once the behavior becomes compulsive, this results in further feelings of shame, interference in interpersonal relationships, and intimacy dysfunction (Coleman, 1987b). Thus the sex compulsivity is a result of intimacy dysfunction and becomes a type of or symptom of intimacy dysfunction.

Sex as a potential agent for a compulsive behavior is naturally alluring. The sexual response cycle causes significant changes in neuroendocrine and body chemistry. These changes can have adrenalin or analgesic-type qualities. The "natural high" from sexual activity can ease pain, help one relax. It can also mask feelings of pain such as low self-esteem. Sex can be used as a "short-cut" to a semblance of positive self-esteem and a feeling of intimacy. During high states of sexual arousal perceptions are changed. These states can be used as an escape from negative or painful perceptions of self and the world. Thus, the potential for developing compulsive or addictive patterns is significant.

This paradigm of the etiology has been most helpful to me clinically in understanding a variety of compulsive behaviors. The other dynamic which seems most evident in the development of sex compulsive behaviors is the background of highly restrictive and conservative attitudes regarding sexuality (see Figure 3) (Coleman, 1986). In response to these environments, my clients have not been able to conform to such restrictive attitudes (usually because they are simply sexual beings). Issues surrounding masturbation, for example, have been commonly traumatic. Many clients report having been severely disciplined for childhood masturbation or carefully watched to prevent masturbation from occurring. As a result of being unable to conform to such restrictions, they cognitively construed themselves as sinful or deviant which resulted in feelings of guilt and shame (and many

```
           Highly Restrictive
          Attitudes on Sexuality
                   │
                   ▼
            Unable to Conform
              to Restrictions
                   │
                   ▼
             Interpret Behavior
            as Sinful or Deviant
                   │
                   ▼
           Feel Guilt and Shame
                   │
                   ▼
                Keep Secrets
                   │
                   ▼
                   Pain
                   │
                   ▼
              Act Compulsively
              to Relieve Pain
```

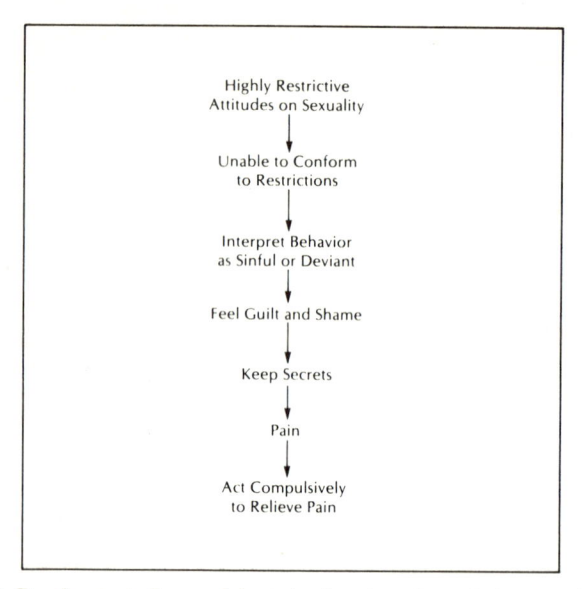

FIGURE 3. Development of compulsive behaviors through restrictive sexual attitudes.

had already developed shame-based personalities even before sexuality had become an issue). In order to alleviate some of the guilt and shame, they became secretive about their sexual behavior to avoid or avert punishment. This whole process, again, produced psychological pain. The individual, then, acted to alleviate the pain through compulsive behavior patterns. Also, as in most obsessive-compulsive disorders, the more the person tried to suppress the impulse, the more compelling it became.

These hypotheses are in need of testing. And this research is now being conducted and hopefully, in the near future, there will be some answers.

RELATIONSHIP TO CHEMICAL DEPENDENCY

It has been noted in the author's clinical practice as well indications from research which is still being conducted and analyzed that chemically dependent individuals have had a higher proportion of sexually compulsive behavior patterns.

It is not surprising that sexual compulsivity is correlated with alcohol or drug abuse and dependency. Many individuals learn how to be sexual while using chemicals as teenagers. When adults socialize, chemicals are often readily available. If individuals go out on a date, the stereotypical format begins with cocktails and ends up with a nightcap and sex. In order to get someone "in the mood," some offer the other a drink. If the goal is to make sex just a little bit better, some will use a drug before making love. Others who are anxious about having sex, a drink or some other drug will help them relax and enjoy. If they are worried about getting an erection, coming too fast, or having an orgasm, they might use the drug more. Some might even resort to purported aphrodisiacs.

Where does this association come from? Two of our society's greatest preoccupations are sex and chemicals. Insofar as they are both preoccupations, they naturally become associated. Marilyn Mason (1983) has described another connection between sex and chemicals: both are linked to romance as our films, novels and other literature reveal. Further, we have another myth that sex and chemicals will lead to romance. Another romantic myth is that not only better living but better sex can be achieved through chemicals. With every myth, there is a bit of reality and a lot of unreality.

Advertising media perpetuate and capitalize on these myths. How many products does sex sell? Many alcohol advertisements that say, "You'll be a sexier person with this type of alcohol." Other advertisements say, "If you want to seduce someone, use this brand of alcohol." We are bombarded daily with these messages in newspapers, magazines, and billboards.

Chemically dependent individuals, growing up in families with intimacy dysfunction, are at high risk for developing unhealthy and distorted attitudes, values and behaviors regarding sex, intimacy, and drugs. For many chemicals are always involved in their sexual behavior. Chemicals stave off feelings of shame and give them the confidence to behave sexually. Some find it is impossible to engage in certain sexual activities without the assistance of chemicals to loosen inhibitions, minimize shame, and give a false sense of security and self-esteem. Chemicals also provide a great excuse for engaging in sexual activities that aren't in one's value system. "I couldn't help it—I was drunk last night." "If I hadn't had that last drink, I would never have done what I did." "I get so horny when I smoke pot." "He(she) got me so drunk, I couldn't say no." Or, the best excuse, "I was so drunk, I don't even remember what happened last night."

Many chemically dependent individuals are stunned in their recovery when their abusive sexual behavior continues without their alibi or justification. They somehow think, "Now that I'm sober, I'll never get myself into those situations again." For some people, that is true. For others, however, their abusive sexual behavior does not change when they stop drinking or using drugs. For some, abusive sexual activity even accelerates.

How would it accelerate and why? First, their alcohol and drug abuse may have been serving as a mechanism to control unwanted sexual urges. Without the control mechanisms, they become overwhelmed with these urges. For others, taking one fix away will necessitate finding another. So a recovering chemically dependent person might say, "Yeah, sobriety is great. I'm having no problems staying sober. And my sex life has never been better. In fact, I'm horny all the time and can't seem to get enough!" This dynamic accounts for how some chemically dependent individuals develop sexual compulsivity after they have sobered up from alcohol or drugs.

Certainly some chemically dependent individuals were or are sexually compulsive during the time of active chemical abuse. Dual or multiple compulsive behaviors are common. The related compulsive behaviors in addition to the chemical dependency, however, are rarely addressed in the treatment of the chemically dependent individual. Somehow, there is a myth in chemical dependency treatment that, "If we purge an individual from chemicals, that all his or her problems will go away." And what's more, "We don't even need to know about these other problems, because they are so often a result of the chemical dependency." The author has worked with clients who have pleaded with their counselors in chemical dependency treatment to do a "first step" on their sexual compulsivity—feeling in some cases that sex is even a stronger "addiction" to them than drugs. The author has found that counselors have discouraged the client to do this because they felt the request was a way of avoiding looking at the primary illness of chemical dependency. There have been a number of clients in this author's clinical practice who have been treated for chemical dependency, when, in fact, their primary compulsion was not primarily alcohol or drugs but certain sexual practices.

Traditionally, chemical dependency treatment centers have had a difficult time talking about sex, period. The link between sexual problems and chemical abuse has been fairly well documented (Coleman, 1982, 1987) yet these problems often go unrecognized and untreated. Aftercare plans of most treatment centers cover just about every aspect of a person's life except sex. Treatment must go beyond the control of drinking or other drug abuse to deal also with family intimacy issues. Upon obtaining sobriety or responsible use, a person is often frozen in insecurity, lacking the skills to develop and express intimacy. Often the chemical abuser is still dependent upon alcohol or other drugs to be sexual or to be intimate, which is why so many seek sexual or intimacy counseling following treatment for chemical abuse or dependency. The chemical use is controlled, but they need something more. We have been training chemical dependency counselors to address more effectively the sexual and intimacy problems of their clients, and, as a result, these issues are being addressed more and more. Things are changing, but it seems we have a long way to go.

The opposite problem is also true. Therapists who have traditionally treated sexual compulsions have often neglected to address the client's chemical abuse problems. These therapists have had a difficult time talking about alcohol and drug use and looking for signs and symptoms of abuse or dependency. They have their own set of blinders. This situation is changing, too, as more and more mental health professionals are being trained in chemical dependency. Many therapists have never had any formal or informal training in chemical dependency. They do not know how to look for signs and symptoms of chemical dependency and rarely even ask questions about chemical use.

CONCLUSION AND SUMMARY

It is important for professionals to recognize the problem of sexual compulsivity and to begin to address this problem in a professional manner. New treatment methods need to be developed and evaluated.

It will be also important to listen and to conduct research on the efforts of the self-help organizations. Professionals tend to have disdain for many self-help organizations because of their lack of professional guidance. And, yet, Alcoholics Anonymous (AA), while not effective with everyone, may be just as effective as traditional, professional treatment programs. In referring clients to these self-help organizations, the author believes that it is important that these groups separate "addictive" forms of sexual expression and "non-addictive" forms. Therefore, it is important that the professional be assured that the particular self-help group's intention is not to purge sexuality from its members.

In addition, it is important that clients be given positive and healthy attitudes regarding sexuality. Unfortunately in some self-help groups, these groups often lack positive messages about sexuality. Those who have suffered pain as a result of their sexuality might be reluctant to give permission to individuals to enjoy sexuality as an important and celebratory part of their lives. There needs to be modelling of healthy sexual expression beyond the control of destructive or abusive patterns of sexual behavior.

Finally, treatment programs of psychotherapists who treat sexual compulsivity need to be knowledgeable about human sexuality as well as personality disorders, addictive disorders, and other forms of mental illness. And, very importantly, the psychotherapists should hold positive and healthy attitudes about their own sexuality and a wide range of sexual expression of other's sexuality. In reviewing the author's hypothesized etiological factors, conservative or restrictive attitudes about sexuality may be one of the important precursors. If treatment simply reinforces these attitudes, then the therapist has contributed to the factors which lead the person to act compulsively. Treatment needs to go beyond control of problematic sexual behavior. First, one must rule out the possibility of the problem being a values conflict between an individual's own expression and societal pressures and if this is a values conflict this should be treated accordingly. If not, treatment again should go beyond the control of sexual behavior and to help the individual develop positive and healthy attitudes regarding sexuality. In the process of treatment, factors which might contribute to compulsive behavior patterns or inhibit healthy sexual expression should be explored: Sexual attitudes, shame about themselves, low self-esteem, lack of personal boundaries or respect for others' psychological boundaries, sex role discomfort, confusion or dysphoria, concerns about sexual orientation, sexual dysfunction, communication skills, dependency patterns in relationships, and means of expressing intimacy.

REFERENCES

Barlow, D. (October 1984). Interview in article by D. Goleman, Some Sexual Behavior Viewed as an Addiction. New York Times, October 16.
Carnes, P. (1983). *Out of the Shadows: Understanding sexual addiction*. Minneapolis, MN: Compcare Publications.
Carnes, P. (1986). Progress in sexual addiction: An addiction perspective. SIECUS Report. Vol. 14(6): 4-6.
Coleman, E. (1982). Family intimacy and chemical abuse: The connection. *Journal of Psychoactive Drugs*. Vol. 14: 153-158.
Coleman, E. (1986). Sexual compulsion vs. sexual addiction: The debate continues. SIECUS Report. Vol. 14(6): 7-11.
Coleman, E. (1987). Chemical dependency and intimacy dysfunction: Inextricably bound. *Journal of Chemical Dependency Treatment*. Vol. 1.
Cushman, L. P. (January-February, 1985). A sexologist's concern. A Special Supplement to the TAOS Newsletter.
Kaufman, G. *Shame: The power of caring*. Cambridge: Shenkman, 1980.
Levine, M. (1985). AIDS and sexual behavior: A panel discussion. Presentation at the Annual Meeting of the Eastern Region of the Society for the Scientific Study of Sex, Philadelphia, PA, April 20.
Mason, M. (1983). Sexuality and fear of intimacy as barriers for recovery for drug dependent women. In B. Reed, C. Bechner & J. Mondanaro (Eds.), *Treatment services for drug dependent women. II*. Washington, DC: U.S. Government Printing Office, U.S. Department of Health and Human Services.
Money, J. (January-February, 1985). Love as Addiction. A Special Supplement to the TAOS Newsletter.
Quadland, M. (November, 1985a) *Overcoming sexual compulsion*. New York Native.
Quadland, M. (1985). Compulsive sexual behavior: Definition of a problem and an approach to treatment. *Journal of Sex and Marital Therapy*, 11(2).
Sharon, R. K. (January-February, 1985). I cannot remain silent. A Special Supplement to the TAOS Newsletter.
Taylor, C. L. (January-February, 1985). A social science perspective of sexual addiction. A Special Supplement to the TAOS Newsletter.

Wedin, R. W. (1985a). *The sexual compulsion movement*. Christopher Street, Issue 88.
Wedin, R. W. (1985b). AIDS and sexual behavior: A panel discussion. Presentation at the Annual Meeting of the Eastern Region of the Society for the Scientific Study of Sex, Philadelphia, PA, April 20.

Treatment of Dependency Disorders in Men: Toward a Balance of Identity and Intimacy

Philip Colgan, MA

SUMMARY. In many male clients struggling with issues of dependency, there are often dysfunctional patterns of recognizing, expressing, and satisfying needs for human contact. This paper presents a conceptual framework of dependency disorders as an organizing principle for understanding such patterns. The discussion will be directed toward the etiology of the patterns, their behavioral manifestations, and effective treatment strategies.

THE PROBLEM: DEPENDENCY DISORDERS

In the present discussion, dependency disorders are defined as dysfunctional patterns utilized by individuals to separately affirm themselves and also to affirm their connections with others. Self affirmation refers to identity, including but not limited to sexual identity. Connections with others refers to intimacy, including but not limited to sexual intimacy. Thus, dependency disorders include both identity disorders and intimacy dysfunctions.

A dependency disorder is not to be confused with the dependent personality disorder as described in DSM-III. Rather, it is a

---

Philip Colgan is in private practice as a licensed psychologist in Minneapolis, MN. He has a clinical appointment at the Program in Human Sexuality, Department of Family Practice and Community Health, Medical School, University of Minnesota.

Requests for reprints can be sent to the author at the Program in Human Sexuality, 2630 University Avenue, S.E., Minneapolis, MN 55414.

The author would like to especially thank Richard Kott, Ann Stefanson, and Geol Weirs for their contributions.

© 1987 by The Haworth Press, Inc. All rights reserved.

distinct, observed clinical phenomenon so named for heuristic purposes. As such, it neither precludes nor replaces DSM-III categories. As a clinical entity, a dependency disorder can be manifested in many categories of symptoms, including eating disorders, alcohol and other drug-dependence, affective disturbances, sexual violence, and other interpersonal violence. While these and many other symptom clusters may appear to be distinct phenomena, the underlying issues are here identified as a dependency disorder. An understanding of dependency disorder can help clinicians utilize effective psychotherapeutic interventions for treatment of the coexisting problems of identity disorders and intimacy dysfunctions.

IDENTITY DISORDER

An identity disorder is defined as inadequate formation and/or development of a personal construct of self-worth. In this definition, a personal construct of self-worth refers to an internal view of oneself as worthwhile. Worthwhile refers to Freud's definition of mental health: to be able to love and to work. Worth is thus defined as being capable of giving and receiving love and having the ability to generate positive contributions to one's own life and the lives of others.

Identity disorders are also characterized by developmental deficits which preclude, interrupt, or distort optimal identity formation and/or development. These deficits, from Erickson (1959), can be grouped under distortions in one's internal frame of reference and distortions in one's external frame of reference. Deficits in internal development include: mistrust of self, doubting one's own perceptions, irrational conformity to the desires of others, and anxiety about acceptability of one's own desires. Deficits in one's external frame of reference include: disregard for the needs of others, excessive needs for control of others, mistrust of others, the inability to share with others, and intolerance of difference.

It appears that these developmental deficits have a common unifying factor. Each represents an identity based on a definition of self as defective in some fundamental way. Kaufman (1974) describes this as shame. Shame, as an organizing principle of the self, eventuates from circumstances where one does not form an identity based on self-worth.

An identity based on a sense of shame represents an identity disorder. In this description, an identity disorder has its basis in undervaluing oneself as a person who can be worthwhile in both love and work. With this internal frame of reference, other beliefs form. Not valuing himself, the man with an identity disorder searches outside himself for value. If what is valuable isn't in the self, it must be outside the self. This represents an external locus of control (Smalley, 1982). Being unable to count on himself for a sense of being worthwhile, the man becomes dependent on reacting to or responding to others' desires as his source of personal value. His over-reliance on others is manifested in intimacy dysfunction.

INTIMACY DYSFUNCTION

Intimacy dysfunction is defined as a pattern of behaviors which precludes a balance of separation and attachment that appears necessary for emotionally satisfying relationships. In this, separation refers to the ability to act in ways which affirm one's worth as an individual. Attachment refers to actions which affirm one's worthwhile connections with others. Thus, separation and attachment refer to the external, behavioral manifestations of one's internal construct of worth.

In this description, "separation" and "attachment" are similar to Bakan's (1966), conceptualization of "agency" and "communion." In the adjective form, to be "agentic" means to assert oneself, to be self-protective, and to define self via one's actions. To be "communal" means to act in such a way that recognizes one's relations to others, to seek and give nurturing, and to define self via one's connections with others. "Agency" then refers to separation. "Communion" refers to attachment.

Intimacy dysfunctions are characterized by patterns of behavior wherein attachment and separation are out of balance. Typically, one with intimacy dysfunction relies on one set of behavior to the exclusion of the other. When this is the case, one either appears to either overvalue individuality (over-separation) or to overvalue human connections (over-attachment). The effects of such an imbalance often involve impaired interpersonal communication, unresolved intrapsychic and interpersonal stress, and dysfunctional behavior patterns designed to cope with the stresses.

Interaction of Identity Disorder and Intimacy Dysfunction

Identity disorders and intimacy dysfunctions interact to form a self-perpetuating cycle. The interaction is best seen in dysfunctional behaviors which appear to be goal directed, yet have built in components which ultimately ensure defeat of goal attainment. For example, the man who routinely uses alcohol to quiet his fears of rejection in social situations certainly appears to express a normal human desire — to have easy discourse with others. But his route for goal attainment requires him to depend on an external agent: alcohol. When this becomes a pattern, he is increasingly left with fewer choices about how to attain his goal. Ultimately, his total lack of choice represents a dependency disorder. Because he can not depend on himself (identity disorder), he depends on alcohol to help him form connections with others (intimacy dysfunction).

Over-Separation and Over-Attachment

Healthy attachment occurs between two people who also separately affirm themselves. This, of course, requires each to have firmly established an identity based on self-worth. When, however, one has not established an identity solidly based on self-worth, he will behave in ways designed to compensate for his lack of self-value. Compensation appears to take forms which indicate an imbalance of attachment and separation. All the compensatory mechanisms appear to share dependence on external agents as the principle which governs behavior.

The example described above serves to illustrate one form of a dysfunctional attachment — to some impersonal external agent, such as a chemical. Other examples of external agents include sex, spending, working out, food, work, or gambling. The compulsive and often ritualized uses of these agents provide diagnostic clues of a dependency disorder for the mental health practitioner.

Sometimes the external agent is another person. Dependence on others for one's positive sense of identity is manifested in two ways: over-attachment and over-separation. Over-attachment involves a pattern of subsuming one's individual identity under the identity of the relationship. The colloquial "you're nobody 'til somebody loves you" says it well (Smalley, 1982). That somebody is always some other person, never oneself. The lack of self-valuing that describes an identity disorder requires connection with an external agent for the man to have any self-definition of worth. For men in this situation, connection is the sole route to identity formation and maintenance.

The second form of unhealthy dependence on others, that of over-separation, involves a pattern of shaping one's identity by reacting to, as opposed to interacting with, others. Other people are used for purposes of contrast or comparison. The man in this situation always appears to come out on top, or he distorts situations to make sure that he thinks he has. The lack of a personal construct of positive self-worth which describes an identity disorder requires external validation for self-worth. For him, this is achieved through contest. If no contest is readily available, he will find one or invent one. For him, distinction from others is the sole route to identity formation and maintenance.

Each form of dependence on an external agent becomes unhealthy when it is used to the exclusion of a balancing force of depending on oneself. This is especially so when the external agent, be it animal, mineral, or vegetable, becomes necessary for establishing and maintaining one's positive sense of self and of well-being. The ability to count on oneself requires an internal frame of reference. This is essential for a positive sense of identity. Reliance on an external agent reveals an external frame of reference. Sole reliance on external agents for a positive sense of identity signals the presence of identity disorder. In close relationships, such identity disorders invariably lead to intimacy dysfunctions.

ETIOLOGY

An understanding of the psychodynamic etiology of dependency disorders will help the clinician work effectively with clients to correct developmental deficits which have interfered with optimal identity formation and development. Toward that end, this section will discuss theoretical and empirical data that address issues of male development, including identity formation, intimacy development, and socialization issues.

Identity Formation: Etiology in the Family

The role of the family in the formation of an identity based on self-worth is best presented here in summary form. Current theorists (e.g., Johnson, 1985) view optimal identity formation as an ongoing internal dialogue between an *apriori* personal construct of self-worth and one's interpretations of others' input. As far as can be known, this begins at birth with primitive and preverbal information processing.

An identity disorder has its roots in the family's responses to the infant at this time. For example, at the same time the infant delights in the discovery of his own uniqueness, he also learns that others do not always share in his delight. Lacking adequate internal cognitive constructs which reinforce his delight, he is at risk for internalizing others' cognitive, affective, and behavioral responses to his emerging self. When those responses are consistently negative, he may prematurely decide that his delight is erroneous. Rather than viewing himself with delight, then, he views himself as wrong or defective in some way. In this way, the pre-existing personal construct of self-worth begins to be deformed into an identity disorder.

INTIMACY DYSFUNCTION: THE FAMILY

How this is reinforced through intimacy dysfunctions can be seen through the family's role in the development of dependency disorders. While the importance of parent/child interactions has been recognized for some time, recent research identifies specific symptoms of dependency disorders linked to family of origin interactions. These include bulimia (Johnson & Flach, 1985), alcoholism (e.g., Wolin et al., 1979), affective disturbances (Cytryn, 1985), physical abuse (Garbarino and Gilliam, 1980) and sexual abuse (Cooper & Cormier, 1982).

These are obvious examples of dysfunctional behavior. But clinical data suggest that more subtle patterns of identity disorders and intimacy dysfunctions can also be transmitted intergenerationally (Colgan & Riebel, 1981). Cohen and Densen-Gerber (1981) report that adults who did not experience nurturing (emotional affirmation) in their own childhoods find it difficult to nurture their children. By contrast, persons whose parents were (emotionally) expressive toward them will be more expressive as adults (Balswick & Avertt, 1977).

Coleman (1983) and Coleman and Colgan (1986), describe a generational cycle of transmission of dependency dynamics. In their model, intimacy dysfunction is taught to children by family members. This is done by the adults' interactions with one another and with the children. The adults' modelling in an environment of experiential learning gives children lasting impressions for how to behave within emotionally close relationships. Through the direct and indirect behavioral expressions of intimacy (and by the absence of these as well), children develop templates for all human interactions. The templates are reinforced by years of repetition of the patterns. And as Adler (1927) suggests, the consequent expectancy effects shape all perceptions of the person's further human interactions.

DEVELOPMENT OF PATTERNS OF OVER-SEPARATION AND OVER-ATTACHMENT

The Family

Johnson (1985) argues that the child who is actively rejected by parents will develop behavioral traits here described as over-separation (unmitigated agency). Further, the child who experiences some form of emotional abandonment by important care givers will try to recoup the loss by behavior patterns here described as over-attachment (unmitigated communion). Block

(1973) reports that boys reared by rejecting fathers and seductive mothers exhibited hypermasculinity, or unmitigated agency (over-separation). Boys reared by emotionally absent fathers and depressed, neurotic mothers exhibited hyperfeminity, or unmitigated communion (over-attachment).

It would appear that young males have ample opportunity for being rejected, leading to over-separation behavior in the adult. For example, male babies are more likely than females to suffer physical abuse (Garbarino & Gilliam, 1980). In the authors' analysis, the rejection often comes from fathers, as more fathers than mothers use physical force to discipline.

Ample opportunity also exists for a boy to be abandoned, leading to over-attachment behavior in the adult. For example, Noller (1978) found that boy-parent dyads had fewer interactions than girl-parent dyads. This study further showed that fathers give more affection to daughters than to sons.

Children are rejected or abandoned by parents who do not act as adequate attachment objects for the subjects. Attachment theorists suggest that anger is an expected response for children reared by such parents (Bowlby, 1975). But boys, as Gleason (1975) reports, are discouraged from verbalizing feelings of anger directly to their fathers and are encouraged to express anger through action, often aggressive action. In the present conceptualization, the action can take the form of over-attachment or over-separation, both of which involve steps taken to control affective expression.

Control of affective expression is further refined by repetition of patterns of rejection or abandonment by parents or other adult care givers. For example, repeated physical or sexual abuse can compound the already existing problems of identity development for the rejected boy. More subtle examples may include disinterest in the boy's activities, except when they are first recognized by outside sources. More apparent, and perhaps more prevalent, is overt criticism of the boy, based on expectations beyond his level of achievement.

Emotional abandonment can continue to occur in the lives of boys reared in homes where the parents' focus is taken up by activities other than the well-being of the child. Examples of such involvement can include the vicissitudes of alcoholism or other addictions, strict adherence to religious principles which don't allow for individual differences, excessive work schedules which are not balanced by "quality time" with the child, or language barriers arising out of cultural differences between the family and the wider society.

RELATIONSHIPS OUTSIDE THE FAMILY: FURTHER DEVELOPMENT OF OVER-ATTACHMENT AND OVER-SEPARATION PATTERNS

The inability to affectively communicate, fostered at home, appears to be reinforced in the wider culture. Miller (1983) argues that the course of socialization teaches the young boy to express emotion via physical aggression, not verbal affective communication. As a result, even when directly questioned about affective states of fear or anxiety, boys are more likely than girls to lie, keeping their feelings secret (Lekarezy & Hill, 1969).

The relationship between affective expressiveness and the development of over-attachment or over-separation behaviors can be better understood by examination of specific patterns of behavior in males. Self-disclosure as a function of positive separation and offering aid to others in distress as a function of positive attachment will be examined here.

One aspect of affective expressiveness is self-disclosure. It is presumed here that the man who values his individuality can affectively express that verbally. Men in general, however, appear to have difficulty with this. For example, Cosby (1973) found that men self-disclose less than women. Rosenfeld (1979) found that men choose not to self-disclose for reasons of maintaining control over themselves and the impressions they give others. Thus, it would appear that men are unlikely to express self-affirmation, or healthy separation, through affective self-disclosure.

Another aspect of affective expressiveness involves giving aid to others. It is assumed here that the man who values his connections with others is able to affectively express that in prosocial behavior. In her excellent review of the literature on sex differences in prosocial behavior, Robinson (1985) concludes that the culture rewards men and women differently for helping those in need. The prevalent view in the literature appears to be that males offer help in tasks where no affective expression is involved. By contrast, many studies suggest that females are more likely to offer help when affective expression (e.g., empathy) is involved. These choices reflect cultural rewards for sex-typed behavior. The differences, interestingly enough, disappear or reverse when anonymity is introduced as a factor in similar studies. Thus, men and women appear to have fewer differences when the cultural expectations for sex-typed behavior are removed. And it would appear that men are likely to express healthy attachment to others only when their affective involvement is kept secret.

If the culture mitigates against males expressing affect verbally regardless of parentage, then it is even more difficult for the male who has been reared by rejecting or abandoning parents to develop integrated identity and intimacy. Clinically, men displaying patterns of over-attachment or over-separation report histories which indicate they learned the "male" rules of behavior too well. What was valued by others became more important than internal cues which contradicted affective inexpressiveness.

The boy with an identity disorder appears to develop a schism between his private *persona* and his public presentation of self. His private truths (statements which reflect his personal construct of worth as it is) and his public truths (statements which reflect what he desires his personal construct of worth to be) lack integration.

The schism is further reinforced through experiential learning in the course of relationships outside the family. Those who view themselves with a personal construct of positive self-worth appear to be able to experiment with new and different behaviors of both attachment and separation. They apparently feel enough freedom to break the sanctions against affective disclosure involving separation and attachment. These continue to shape or reinforce his positive view of the self. Others, lacking this essential base, act to conceal their deficits in order to experiment with separation and attachment. The former group continues to grow, expand, and refine healthy separation and attachment behavior. The latter group interrupts this process of learning. They apparently need to protect themselves from reexperiencing the rejection or abandonment experienced as a child. The principal difference between the two groups appears to be related to their use of opportunities for affective expressiveness.

More definite conclusions await empirical investigation. Further exploration of these issues will give both clinicians and clients a better understanding of the evolution of dysfunctional patterns of satisfying needs for both separation and attachment observed in male clients.

PATTERNS OF DEPENDENCY DISORDERS IN ADULT RELATIONSHIPS

An identity disorder has been defined as the inadequate development of a personal construct of self-worth. How men reinforce this identity in intimacy dysfunctions within adult relationships is the focus of this section. The discussion is intended to help the clinician recognize possible problem areas and find direction for psychotherapeutic intervention with men displaying these patterns.

Cognitive, Affective, and Behavioral Components

Patterns involving over-separation and/or over-attachment can be identified by affective, behavioral, and cognitive components. See Table A.

From the previous discussion, it appears that the man who has been actively rejected by his parents will display over-separation patterns. The man who has experienced an interruption of healthy attachment with parents will respond in adulthood with patterns of over-attachment. In the adult, both patterns are reactionary attempts to maintain affective homeostasis. Men may rely on one pattern or the other until fatigue and mounting tension require them to do something different. Often, doing something different means choosing the less-frequently used coping pattern. Therefore, in one man, it is clinically usual to observe periodic swings from over-attachment to over-separation. The shifts often happen without warning.

Consequently, he is puzzled by his own feelings, thoughts, and behaviors as he goes ricocheting through his days. He is buffeted by his deep desire to both be himself and to fit into a

216 CHEMICAL DEPENDENCY AND INTIMACY DYSFUNCTION

Table A

OVER-SEPARATION	OVER-ATTACHMENT
Feelings	
fears smothering	fears abandonment
self controlled	out of control
indifferent	needy/burdened
unsafe with others	unsafe alone
trapped	shut out
numb	desperate
Behaviors	
self protective	self sacrificing
controls others	pleases others
acts to guard feelings	acts contrary to feelings
denies	explains
compulsively independent	compulsively dependent
Thoughts	
"You're not good enough."	"I'm not good enough."
"They want so much."	"I want so little."
"They give so little."	"I give so much."
"I'm ambivalent."	"You don't care."
"If only they would..."	"What am I doing wrong?"
"I am a rock."	"I'm nobody without you."
"You should be grateful."	"I'm so unappreciated."
PHILIP COLGAN, M.A.	CHEMICAL DEPENDENCY and
copyright 1985	FAMILY INTIMACY

society where "All men are created equal" but "May the best man win."

THE CYCLE OF OVER-SEPARATION

Men who operate in over-separation patterns strive to be independent of others at all costs. This is to avoid a repetition of the rejection experienced as an infant. When he was initially rejected, the development of his personal construct of self-worth was distorted by his need for protection from the perceived attack. Protection, as an infant, meant pulling back from the threat of involvement with other people. He consequently experiences boyhood activities as challenges to his defensive and offensive abilities. Winning becomes paramount. So as a child, he doesn't learn how to share, or be emotionally involved except to celebrate victory over a vanquished attacker.

As an adult, he continues to need independence to feel worthwhile. The only hope of happiness is to protect himself from losing. He's able to rationalize any failures. In order to win, he watches others carefully so that he engages only when winning is assured.

At the same time, however, his internal thoughts remind him of his desire to rest and have easy interactions with others. But to have any needs for emotional connection with others means panic for him. It bodes failure, as he has not learned how to be intimate. Consequently, to control these normal human responses, he works to satisfy them in ways that, although indirect, are controllable.

These take the form of external agents. The agents substitute for human connection. Or they offer access to human connection while at the same time camouflaging his deep needs for acceptance. The specific forms can include sex, gambling, spending, food, work, physical fitness programs, or alcohol or other drugs. The relief from the anxiety of being alone and wanting connection is real. The only problem is that it is temporary. Sometimes, the time lapse between the need and the substitution becomes so short that he no longer recognizes his emotional needs. Or he denies them. And while the substitutions are dependable at first, in time they too start to fail him and depression may set in.

In his one-to-one relationships, he appears to have two choices: to lead or be a loner. Leading means making sure he's never at fault. Being a loner absolutely assures him he can't lose. When he couples, he often seeks someone who initially appears to need nothing from him, or needs only that which he gives. In fact, his choice is often someone who admires his independence and strength. In time, however, he increasingly feels pressure to also be emotionally responsive. Lacking the skills for this, he often retreats into numbness. He becomes more and more unaware of both his own needs and the needs of people near him. Repeated requests for emotional connection will eventually be met with intense bursts of anger which mask his helplessness. See Figure 1.

The internal, and probably unconscious, litany describing his personal construct of self-worth may sound something like this:

THE INTERNAL LITANY OF OVER-SEPARATION:
HEROES DON'T NEED. so I
 FAKE IT.   and
  TRY HARDER.   because
   LIFE IS A TEST.   that
    I SHOULD . . .   always
     BE IN CONTROL.   of so that I
      NEVER FAIL.

THE CYCLE OF OVER-ATTACHMENT

Men who operate in patterns of over-attachment strive to connect with others at all costs. This is to avoid a repetition of the abandonment experienced as an infant. When he was initially abandoned, the development of his personal construct of self-worth was interrupted. With his primitive information processing system, it appears that the infant attributes the abandonment to some unidentified personal failure. He consequently experiences failure during childhood and adolescence as proof of his unwor-

CYCLE OF OVER-SEPARATION

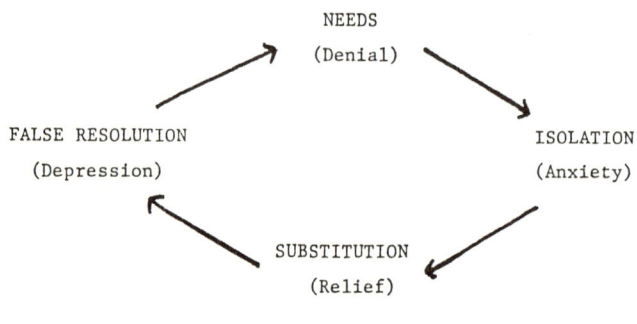

```
                    NEEDS
                   (Denial)

   FALSE RESOLUTION              ISOLATION
     (Depression)                 (Anxiety)

                 SUBSTITUTION
                   (Relief)
```

Figure 1

thiness. From his point of view, when other boys try on the ways of the heroes, they are greeted with enthusiasm and encouragement. When he tries on the ways of heroes, he is greeted with ridicule, derision, and humiliation. As a child, then, he doesn't learn to trust himself and be confident in his abilities alone.

As an adult he needs to be attached to someone else to feel worthwhile. The only hope of happiness is to fit in — to do what others tell him, to please them, to "do the right thing." His sense of self-worth comes from his ability to accommodate others. To accommodate others, he watches them carefully to know in advance how to behave in order to be included.

At the same time, however, his internal thoughts remind him of his unworthiness. His fear is that others will discover this. When they do, they will surely leave him. His terror has its roots in his unconscious sense of having once been good enough to receive love, but somewhere having made a fatal mistake which makes him forever unlovable.

In his adult relationships, he may have a history of joining organized groups in a search for his positive identity. Sometimes he may find a fit. Other times, and more often, he takes on the rituals and practices of the group even if they don't fit. This leaves him puzzled: if the group serves everybody else's needs, why doesn't it serve his? His internal sentence is: "What's wrong with me?"

In his one-to-one relationships, he quite sincerely seeks a partner who will accept him. But his search usually stops with the first person who expresses interest, even if the two are ill-matched. In fact, he often chooses someone who appears to need exactly what he can give: his attention. In some cases, he picks someone who is either unwilling or unable to return this.

Even if the partner can be emotionally responsive, he is too busy "giving" to notice. He tries to do everything right, but because he never fully accepts the gifts of others, an empty feeling of discomfort and discouragement creeps in. Still, he tries his best to make the relationship work by giving time, energy, money, sex — anything his partner wants. But never being a recipient, he feels increasingly burdened — being together is exhausting, but the thought of being alone is terrifying. Not allowing himself to receive, he nonetheless blames his partner for his lack of satisfaction. This external focus staves off his growing internal despair.

As the cycle continues, his energy may give out. Or his partner may become dissatisfied by his inability to receive. Or his constant attention becomes interpreted as clinging and smothering. In any case, abandonment by the partner in even the smallest ways will be interpreted as his personal failure. His sense of exposure leaves him feeling thoroughly ashamed. At that point his intense needs for connection, coupled with his inability to separately affirm himself, bring on a sense of desperation. (See Figure 2.)

TREATMENT CONSIDERATIONS

In the psychotherapeutic treatment of men displaying imbalance in patterns of attachment and separation, the goal becomes that of creating balance. For men using over-separation, this will mean learning new skills which help him incorporate attachment behavior. For men using over-attachment, this will mean learning new skills which help him incorporate separation behavior. Because each pattern of imbalance rests on a faulty conception of the self, redevelopment of a personal construct of positive self-worth is a necessary first step.

Toward that, it is important for the clinician to keep in mind that the goals of the dysfunctional patterns are, in themselves, life-enhancing for the individual. While routes chosen for goal attainment are the targets of intervention, respect for the client's innate desires to both affirm himself separately and affirm himself in relation to others is never under question.

Sometimes the goals in over-separation are sedative, quieting anxiety. In other cases, the goals are directed toward stimulation, to give him a greater sense of interacting with life. The goals are entirely reasonable. The goals of over-attachment are, eminently acceptable as well — to form a stable and lasting bond with another human being. Dissatisfaction comes from the paths described for reaching the goals.

The paths are unsatisfying when identity and intimacy are confused. Depending solely on external agents for positive personal

CYCLE OF OVER-ATTACHMENT

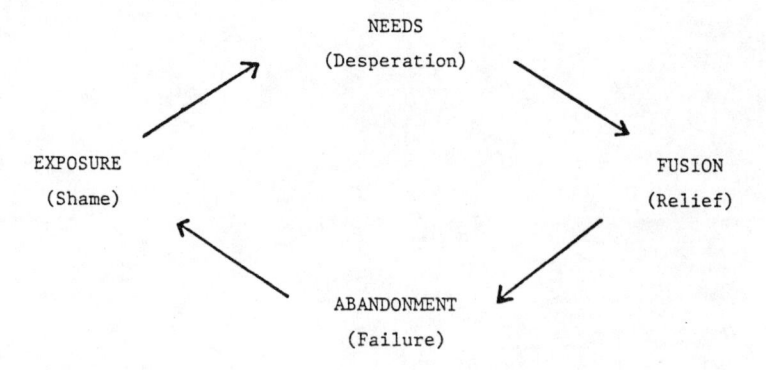

```
                     NEEDS
                  (Desperation)
          ↗                      ↘
EXPOSURE                              FUSION
 (Shame)                              (Relief)
          ↖                      ↙
                  ABANDONMENT
                    (Failure)
```

The internal, and probably unconscious, litany describing his personal construct of worth may sound something like this:

THE INTERNAL LITANY OF OVER-ATTACHMENT

I'M NO HERO ... and

    I NEED ...   so I

        DO EVERYTHING. to

            PLEASE OTHERS. and make

                PEACE AT ANY PRICE. otherwise

                    I WILL LOSE YOU. and, you see,

                        I'M NOBODY WITHOUT YOU.

Figure 2

constructs of self-worth ensures the loss of that goals as well as the loss of the desired intimate connection.

A model for integrating healthy separation and attachment is presented in Figure 3. The model rests on the individual's internal belief that he is worthy of giving and receiving love, and that he is able to both generate output and respond to others' input in the form of positive contributions to life. Or more simply put: to find satisfaction in both love and work.

Inherent in this is the ability to recognize, express, and satisfy

A MODEL FOR IDENTITY AND INTIMACY

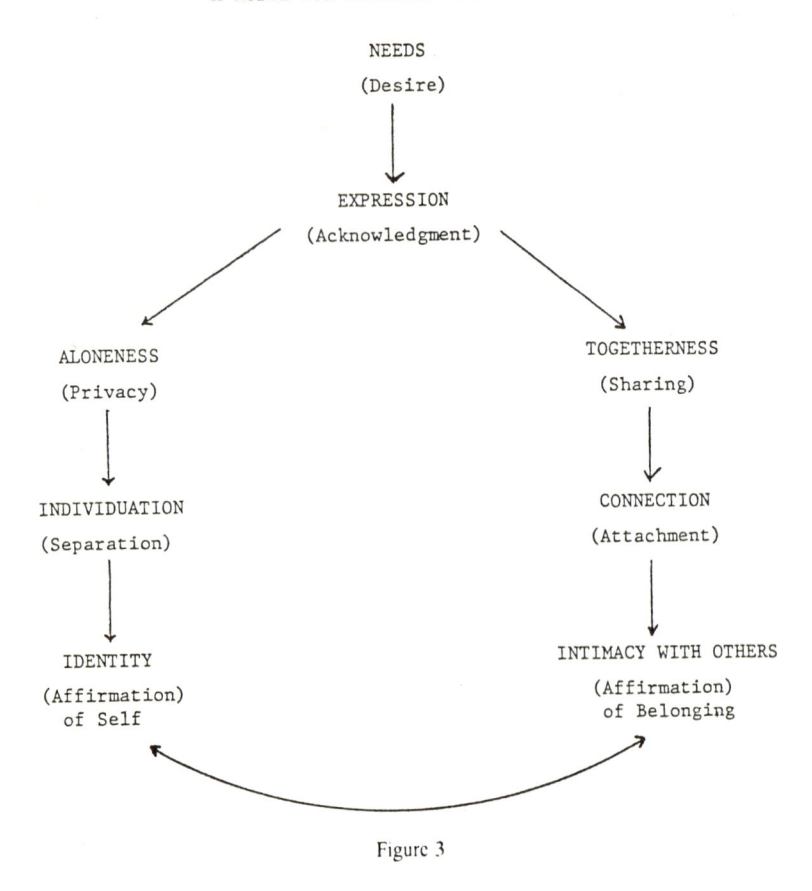

```
                    NEEDS
                   (Desire)
                      |
                      v
                  EXPRESSION
              (Acknowledgment)
              /              \
             v                v
        ALONENESS         TOGETHERNESS
        (Privacy)          (Sharing)
            |                  |
            v                  v
       INDIVIDUATION        CONNECTION
       (Separation)        (Attachment)
            |                  |
            v                  v
         IDENTITY       INTIMACY WITH OTHERS
       (Affirmation)      (Affirmation)
         of Self           of Belonging
              <----------->
```

Figure 3

his needs for both separation and attachment. When the model is operative, he is able to both affirm himself as an individual and affirm his connections with others. Further, when the two are in balance, they interact to reinforce one another.

IDENTITY DEVELOPMENT

The first step in the redevelopment of a personal construct of positive worth involves removal of the negative self-evaluation prematurely formed by one who was rejected or abandoned by parents during infancy. This means redeveloping the capacity to observe one's thoughts, feelings, behaviors, and their consequences without the debilitating judgment inherent in shame (Smalley & Coleman, 1987). Behaviorally, this takes the form of collecting data about oneself with the cold eye of a scientist who reserves judgment until all observations are made.

With this, the client can begin to notice how he currently behaves in ways which maximize separation or attachment. He may want to collect additional data from those he interacts with at home, in school, on the job, or during leisure activities. Personality or vocational tests supplied by the therapist can be used to augment his data supply.

The second step involves increasing one's options for behavior choices in any given situation. Toward this end, the client is encouraged to explore the world as an infant would: with experimentation through trial and error. As he begins to experiment, the client can collect new data about how the options he has developed help him attain satisfying separation or attachment. What distinguishes this process from that which he experienced in infancy is the ability to return to an increasingly solid base of self-worth, regardless of the success or failure of his choices.

As the client gathers new data about his affective and behavioral choices, he will also require new cognitive input. Learning in the forms of bibliotherapy, attendance at classes devoted to human development (e.g., interpersonal communication skills), and discussion of new ideas with other people can all aid in this step.

INTIMACY

While the client collects data and explores new options, the therapist can play a vital role in the client's recovery. By observation of himself, the client will begin to understand the role of the dysfunctional behavior patterns in protecting him from expressing his needs for both separation and attachment. The value of the therapist is in responding to the client with cognitive interest and affective support.

Understandably, the client will experience the affective response to the early rejection or abandonment as he recognizes his needs. The therapist can assume the crucial role of attending to the client in the way he wishes his parents had — with the support of wisdom from a long-range and seasoned perspective, with encouragement in experimentation, and with unquestioning acceptance in the face of failure.

In this way, the therapist provides the basis for healthy intimacy expression by teaching the client to recognize and verbally express the affective responses which arise. Sometimes the teaching is directive, by labelling the affect observed. At other times, the client is encouraged to monitor physiological changes which signal the presence of affective responses. In these ways, the client learns to monitor and label his own affective responses.

Recognition and verbal expression of affect corrects the developmental deficits revealed by patterns of over-attachment and over-separation. Identification of needs leads to greater positive self-recognition (separation) (Smalley, 1982). Expression of the needs to an accepting outsider forms the interpersonal link for affirmation of self in connection with others (attachment) (Kaufman, 1974).

A second important function of the therapist in this process is in helping the client learn how to steer himself toward behaviors which reinforce his capacity for positive identity and intimacy, rather than reinforce the dysfunctional patterns so well learned. The concept of parenting which is both "firm and tolerant" (Erickson, 1959) is pertinent here. In this regard, the client is taught to recognize that desires to engage in dysfunctional behavior are very likely the outgrowth of the anxiety which reappears with recognition of needs. While as an infant, the client was in reality helpless to meet his needs. Now, as an adult, he has other options. Consequently, desires to return to behavior patterns which are no longer useful are met with understanding of the motivation (toleration). But actions which work toward behavior change despite the anxiety are encouraged (firmness).

IDENTITY AND INTIMACY

Men who have relied on patterns of over-separation will be able to risk interpersonal rejection when they know they will not emotionally reject themselves. Further, as they discover that the therapist will neither overwhelm them emotionally, nor shame them for their tenderness, they can continue to explore their needs for attachment. Men who have relied on patterns of over-attachment will be able to risk relying on themselves when they know the therapist will not emotionally abandon them as they become increasingly separate. Further, as they discover that the therapist will not shame them for their desire for independence, they can incorporate the neglected behavior choices.

When the client affectively learns that recognition and expression of needs will not lead to rejection or abandonment of him as an individual, he can begin to experiment with new behavior in relationships outside of therapy. Self-help support groups (such as Alcoholics Anonymous, Alanon, etc.) offer excellent opportunities for this. In them he can have greater assurance that others will understand his process and help him achieve more effective routes for attaining both his personal and interpersonal goals.

Often, clients recognize that the wounds of the past rejection or abandonment require redressing. For some, this means direct confrontation with the parent(s). This can be accomplished either in family therapy where the parent(s) are actively involved, or outside the therapy relationship. In either case, it appears that the parents' willingness to acknowledge the parenting mistakes often helps relieve the pent up affect toward the rejection or abandonment. From this point, affective forgiveness, rather than cognitive "understanding" can help all involved achieve the healthy attachment and separation missed during the client's infancy.

In other cases, circumstances force the client to redress the past in the absence of the parent(s). This presents a greater clinical challenge. Nonetheless the client can move through the delayed affective response via fantasy and imagery with the guidance of the therapist.

Further involvement of the therapist in working with the client and his relationships will be indicated as he attempts new behavior in his close relationships. Often, the disruptive effects of change lead to the necessity of addressing changes in marital and other current family relationships. Toward this, the client may desire to include his partner in the therapy (if this is not already the case). This positive step is effective when the therapist also establishes an independent therapeutic alliance with the partner. When this is not possible, referral to another therapist for the couple's therapy may be indicated.

In either case, couple's or family treatment is effective for swiftly redressing unexpressed affect associated with events in the relationship's history. In addition, clients can experiment with riskier separation and attachment behavior in the emotionally safe environment of therapy.

Therapy is terminated by mutual consent when the client is able to more consistently use his new skills in intimacy functioning, based on a positive personal construct of self-worth. This is indicated when he is able to respond to himself with nonjudgmental recognition of needs for both separation and attachment, to express these without shame, and to behaviorally satisfy them in ways that are both firm and tolerant.

Identity reformation and intimacy functioning are not static products, but rather are components of an ongoing process of discovery and experience. As such, clients may sometimes "take a break" from therapy to experience their growth. The therapist who can offer clients an "open door" for resuming the therapy at a later date can relieve them from reexperiencing rejection or abandonment in unhealthy ways.

SUMMARY

Through the process of identity reformation, the client relies on the therapist for responses which redevelop a personal construct of self-worth (separation). In this process, the therapist also helps the client learn new skills for expressing needs for connection (attachment). The client gradually learns to respond to himself with positive affirmation (separation) in the presence of the therapist. This provides the basis for conscious verbal expression and behavioral steps which affirm his relationships and others (attachment).

REFERENCES

Adler, A. (1927). *Understanding human nature*. Trans. W. B. Wolfe. New York: Greenberg Publishers, Inc.
Bakan, D. (1966). *The duality of human existence*. Chicago: Rand McNally.
Balswich, J. & Avertt, C. P. (1977). Differences in expressiveness: Gender, interpersonal orientation, and perceived parental expressiveness as contributing factors. *Journal of Marriage and the Family, 38*, 121-127.

Block, J. H. (1973, June). Conceptions of sex role: Some cross-cultural and longitudinal perspectives. *American Psychologist*, 512-526.

Bowlby, J. (1975). Attachment theory, separation anxiety, and mourning. In A. Silvano (Ed.), *The American handbook of psychiatry* (Vol. 6, pp. 292-309). New York: Basic Books.

Cohen, F. & Densen-Gerber, J. (1982). A study of the relationship between child abuse and drug addiction in 178 patients: Preliminary results. *Child Abuse and Neglect*, 6, 383-387.

Coleman, E. (1983). Sexuality and the alcoholic family: Effects of chemical dependence and co-dependence upon individual family members. In Golding, P. (Ed.), *Alcoholism: Analysis of a World-Wide Problem*. Lancaster, England: MTP Press Limited.

Coleman, E. & Colgan, P. (1986). Boundary inadequacy in drug dependent families. *Journal of Psychoactive Drugs*, *18*, 21-30.

Colgan, P. & Riebel, J. (1981). *Sexuality education for foster parents*. Minneapolis: University of Minnesota.

Cooper, I. & Cormier, B. (1982). Inter-generational transmission of incest. *Canadian Journal of Psychiatry*, *27*, 231-235.

Cosby, P. C. (1973). Self disclosure: A literature review. *Psychological Bulletin*, 79(2), 73-91.

Cytryn, L., McKnew, D., Zahn-Waxler, C., Radke-Yarrow, M., Gaensbauer, T., Harmon, R. & Lamour, M. (1984, February). A developmental view of affective disturbances in the children of affectively ill parents. *American Journal of Psychiatry*, *141*(2), 219-222.

Erikson, E. (1959). *Identity and the life cycle*. New York: W. W. Norton.

Garbarino, J. & Gilliam, G. (1980). *Understanding abusive families*. Lexington, MA: Lexington Books.

Gleason, J. B. (1975). Fathers and other strangers: Men's speech to young children. In D. P. Dato (Ed.), *Georgetown University roundtable on language and linguistics. Developmental theory and applications*. Washington, DC: Georgetown University Press.

Johnson, C. & Flach, A. (1985, November). Family characteristics of 105 patients with bulimia. *American Journal of Psychiatry*, *142*(11).

Johnson, S. (1985). *Characterological transformation: The hard work miracle*. New York: W. W. Norton.

Kaufman, G. (1974). The meaning of shame: Toward a self-affirming identity. *Journal of Counseling Psychology*, *21*(6), 568-574.

Lakarczyk, D. T. & Hill, K. T. (1969). Self esteem, test anxiety, stress, and verbal learning. *Developmental Psychology*, *1*, 147-154.

Miller, J. B. (1983). The construction of anger in women and men. *Works in Progress* #83-01. Wellesley, MA: Wellesley College.

Noller, P. (1978). Sex differences in the socialization of affectionate expression. *Developmental Psychology*, *14*(3), 317-319.

Robinson, J. (1985). *Sex differences in prosocial behavior: A reexamination*. Unpublished Manuscript: University of Minnesota.

Rosenfeld, L. B. (1979). Self disclosure avoidance: Why am I afraid to tell you who I am? *Communication Monographs*, *46*, 63-74.

Smalley, S. (1982). *Co-dependency: An introduction*. New Brighton, MN: SBS Publications.

Smalley, S. & Coleman, E. (1987, in press).

Wolin, S., Beannett, L. & Noonan, D. (1979, April). Family rituals and the recurrence of alcoholism over generations. *American Journal of Psychiatry*, *136*(4B), 589-593.

Treating Intimacy Dysfunctions in Dyadic Relationships Among Chemically Dependent and Codependent Clients

Sondra Smalley, MA
Eli Coleman, PhD

SUMMARY. When treating intimacy dysfunctions in chemically dependent and codependent relationships, the therapist must focus on resolution of the codependency patterns in order to be successful. Codependency patterns contain several traits (characteristics) or a single state (a fundamental relationship). This paper describes a treatment method which addresses the intimacy dysfunctions among dyadic relationships that display codependency traits. Through three stages of treatment, the therapist can help clients see patterns of their relationships, learn that these patterns are learned and can be unlearned, and that the individual can gain personal power and inner resources. The results of this therapeutic approach leads to healthy intimacy expression based upon individuation of the clients rather than on compulsive codependent patterns.

Problems related to intimacy expression, sexual activity, bonding, and connecting affect most people some of the time.

Sondra Smalley is a licensed psychologist in private practice in New Brighton, MN and is a clinical faculty member of the Program in Human Sexuality, Department of Family Practice and Community Health, Medical School, University of Minnesota.

Dr. Coleman is Associate Director and Associate Professor at the Program in Human Sexuality.

Requests for reprints may be sent to Sondra Smalley, 185 Windsor Court, New Brighton, MN 55112.

The authors would like to thank Orlo Otteson for his editorial assistance in preparing this manuscript.

© 1987 by The Haworth Press, Inc. All rights reserved.

But add chemical dependency and codependency and the complexity of all these problems increases. Chemical dependency and codependency are inextricably bound with intimacy dysfunction (Coleman, 1987). For many years, it has been well known that the relationships of chemically dependent individuals have been difficult, strained or destructive. These relationships include marital, relational, sexual, parent-child, friendship, work, and spiritual relationships. Marital relationships among chemically dependent and codependent persons are often conflictual. Separation and divorce threats are common. Partners are often engaged in a perpetual battle for control and show an inability to engage in effective communication. They have difficulty expressing affection and anger in constructive ways. Sexual incompatibility is common and is evidenced by sexual dysfunction, sexual disinterest, inequality of sexual expectations, disagreements about the types of sexual activities, and/or an inability to be sexual without chemicals. The root of many of these problems is an intimacy dysfunction. Many of the behaviors stem from either a frustrating attempt to remain non-intimate or a frustrated and desperate struggle to create intimacy. When the problem is traced back further, there is frequently evidence of chemical dependency coupled with intimacy dysfunction in the family of origin.

This is not to say that chemical dependency is the cause of all troubles in a dyadic relationship. The authors believe that concerns with intimacy in chemically dependent and codependent relationships are often systemic and might have occurred without the dynamics of chemical dependency. But the dynamics of intimacy dysfunction and chemical dependency increase the severity of other problems in the dyadic relationship. It is also the authors contention that many of the problems of intimacy and chemical dependency are related to codependency patterns. Thus, when treating intimacy dysfunctions in chemically dependent and codependent relationships, the therapist must focus on resolution of the codependency patterns in order for treatment to be successful (Smalley, 1982).

Addressing codependency is a challenge and a problem that the authors are attempting to both describe and to change. We are aware that these efforts are pioneering. One of the struggles is the integration of both the intrapsychic focus with the interactional one. As the Group for the Advancement of Psychiatry states (1970; 565-6):

> In order that we arrive at a mature integration and a resulting "elegant" theory of close relationships, both component fields (individual personality dynamics and multipersonal systems notions) have to develop conceptually as well as methodologically . . .

Codependency can be defined as an easily identifiable (overt) or carefully disguised (covert) learned pattern of exaggerated dependency and extreme and painful external validation, with resulting identity confusion. The pattern can contain several traits (characteristics) or a single state (a fundamental relationship interaction). When evaluating and treating clients, it is important to keep this distinction in patterns in mind and to make this differential assessment.

OVERT AND COVERT FORMS OF CODEPENDENCY

The complexity increases when the codependent person presents himself or herself as either compulsively dependent or as compulsively independent. The same client may be both vulnerably dependent and defiantly independent and swing back and forth between these two stances. Some of these divergent characteristics can be seen in Table 1.

Table 1

The Stances of the Codependent Person

Compulsive Dependence	*Compulsively Independent*
Feels out of control	Feels in control
Feels "needy"	Denies needs
High need for nurturing	High need for achievement
Compliant	Defensive
Passive	Avoidant

With the characteristics in the left column, the psychological focus is external—always outside. From time to time, this kind of person becomes worn or fearful and swings into a defensive posture that is still externally focused. This experience is usually followed by feelings of guilt for being "non-caring," and the individual swings back to a position of non-clarified boundaries. Both stances are characterized by anxiety, which produces hypervigilant external focus.

Most codependent clients go from one stance to another, which results in an inability to focus on self or to develop individual differentiation. These individuals may present themselves in one or another stance or be constantly vacillating between the two. Some clients can take either stance in different areas of their lives. For example, some clients are compulsively independent in the areas of work and community life and compulsively dependent in intimate relationships. One might find a client who is compulsively independent on his/her job and values autonomy and "being able to do things for oneself without any help from anyone else" but who is compulsively dependent in his/her personal life—holding on to relationships that are destructive because of "not being able to be alone."

THE UNDERLYING BELIEFS OF CODEPENDENCY

The compulsively independent/dependent person believes that one must be always perfect. When these individuals fail to meet that impossible standard, they experience and communicate great feelings of shame. To these clients, differentiation and autonomy may mean disintegration. And, cohesion and intimacy may also mean disintegration. Receiving represents selfishness. These beliefs must be addressed by the therapist in order for change.

The degree of resistance of a client to addressing their identity and intimacy issues seems proportional to the client's degree of anxiety. Often the individuation process is perceived by the client as trauma: "I feel I'd be nothing if I was not in a relationship." This compulsively dependent stance is one of personal emptiness and self-alienation. On the other hand, the intimacy process may also be perceived as trauma: "I feel I'll be smothered if I get too close." This compulsively independent stance is also one of emptiness and self-alienation.

There is a dual fear in these clients; merging and abandonment (Mowrer, 1961). They may tend to have one of these fears predominantly as a result of past relationship histories. Acculturation influences these fears as well. Traditional sex-roles suggest that females should fear abandonment and males fear merging (the "reluctant bride-groom" and the "designing woman"). In our experience, however, the differences seem more related to sex-role stereotypes than reality.

CHARACTERISTICS OF CODEPENDENCY

Some of the characteristics of codependency are: (1) high tolerance for inappropriate behavior countered by tolerance breaks; (2) great importance given to external validation; (3) belief that caring must mean being "responsible for" those one cares about rather than being "responsible to"; (4) a tendency to present oneself as always adult, "put together," "surface maturity"; (5) confusion about intimate and sexual roles; (6) "spectatoring" — observing another's performance and not one's own; (7) distorting relationships either by maximizing or minimizing similarities and differences, often displaying either pseudo-hostility or pseudo-mutuality; (8) the inability to get one's dependency needs met; (9) boundary inadequacy (Coleman and Colgan, 1986); and (10) unrealistic expectations of self and others.

IS THIS PATTERN A DISEASE OR A PATTERN?

The authors believe that codependency is a set of learned behavioral, emotional, and attitudinal patterns that can be either personality traits or personality disorders. In either case, this pattern is not a primary disease. These are important distinctions because of the potential aetrogenic effects of an inaccurate labeling process.

In the case of personality traits of codependency, the individual has enduring patterns of perceiving and thinking about others and oneself. These traits are exhibited in important social contexts. This is in keeping with the definition of personality traits as defined in the Diagnostic and Statistical Manual of the American Psychiatric Association (DSM-III). In the case of personality disorders of codependency, the individual is seen as having inflexible and maladaptive behaviors that cause either significant impairment or subjective distress.

The treatment method outlined in this paper addresses the problem of intimacy dysfunctions among dyadic relationships that display codependency traits. These traits may vary in intensity and duration, depending on individual variations and past learning histories. It is the view of the authors that the treatment of codependency disorders would differ. (For a more thorough discussion of the distinction of codependency as a disease, personality disorder or trait, see Gierymski and Williams, 1986 and Cermak, 1986.)

TREATMENT STRATEGIES

What strategies seem useful in treating codependent clients? Since all interaction and therapy take place in the "potential space" (Davis & Wallenbridge, 1981), boundary issues are all important from the beginning. Clients need to be temporarily protected from impingement of their boundary system by others as well as themselves. Usually, specific permission must be given to the client to explore and to try on new reactions (e.g., not doing assignments, compulsively doing assignments, being passive, being aggressive). It is important to "let them be."

The assumptions of this treatment model are that self-awareness is: (1) fostered by information about codependent patterns; (2) best begun in an environment that is non-threatening so that boundaries are preserved; and (3) a process of encouraging gentle self-confrontation followed gradually with firmer self-confrontation.

The authors contend that treatment must change from the old notion that people in primary relationships with chemically dependent individuals are people who need: understanding of the nature of the illness of chemical dependency; understanding of the characteristics and dynamics of chemically dependent individuals; helping them learn communication skills; learning negotiation skills; directing of their feelings toward their partner; and learning to state their desires assertively in their relationship. In fact, we believe we have often encouraged the codependency with these focuses.

The authors do not think the immediate focus on the relationship must be the primary approach. The authors believe the task is, first, not to assume that the dependent relationship will improve by focusing on the dependent relationship, even though clients often insist on this approach. Most individuals first need to come to some clarification about their own patterns, boundaries, and history—apart from all present relational issues.

Perhaps an individual might discover some problems that need more specific treatment, such as an inability to be intimate because of past traumatic experiences with intimacy (e.g., incest, physical abuse, rape, or other forms of boundary invasion). Or an individual may recognize discomfort with his or her own sexual identity—gender identity, sex-role identity, or sexual orientation identity. This sexual identity confusion or discomfort can certainly pose a barrier to intimacy. Finally, the individual may discover other compulsive behavior patterns other than chemicals or codependency. Work, food, and sex compulsivity are commonly seen. These other compulsive behaviors need to be addressed. Each of these also result in intimacy dysfunction.

STAGE ONE—FOCUSING ON IDENTITY

When a couple with codependent traits or states come into therapy to resolve intimacy and sexual concerns, the authors begin to focus initially on each individual's identity in the dyadic relationship. The goal of this stage of therapy is to get the client to become aware of his or her pattern of codependency. A protective stance toward the "potential space" of even the therapy situation and the client's own "inner space" is first essential. Codependent clients do not know how they can protect their own "inner space," and they often blur their boundaries in most interactions. Thus the client is allowed to "be"—without direction or reaction. This stage of therapy can be accomplished in individual therapy or group therapy. These therapy sessions are designed to allow the codependent client to be alone while in other's presence. The environment is manipulated rather than the client responses or behaviors.

In the case of group therapy for the individuals in the dyadic relationship, the design of these groups includes the following dimensions:

1. The goal of individuation is made clear, and non-emphasis on "we-ness" is also stated. (In the authors' experience this is usually met with client approval; and clients share accounts of previous therapy experiences in which they had become so involved in others' dilemmas and solutions that again they somehow avoided consistent self-observation.)
2. Many of the traditional chemical dependency family treatment methods neglect this stage. Traditionally, treatment encourages a "group feeling" — a bridging between the participants and views building these relationships in group as a useful therapeutic technique. But in working with clients with codependency, the authors discourage this kind of interaction. Group participants are encouraged instead to focus on themselves, not on others.
3. In groups, the analogy of "parallel play" is used as a model of interaction. This play may be observed in pre-schoolers who contentedly play side-by-side aware of each other's presence but primarily focused on their own mud pies. As the treatment process continues, this format is gradually changed to encourage some bridging with other participants, with an emphasis on sharing similar relational patterns.

In both individual and group therapies, the authors encourage intensive journal writing as an important treatment method. The client is encouraged to buy a hard-bound book and is given the following rules:

1. This is to be written to yourself to be read five years from now. It is a record of your self-observations and can include if you wish, grocery lists, budget, lists of work to do, anthropological data, etc.
2. It is extremely important that this record be viewed as totally private — to be read by no one. Sometimes a codepen-

dent individual will have great difficulty determining how to ensure the book's privacy. Of course, this elicits the inherent boundary issues of most codependent individuals (Here George Herbert Mead's, 1962, concept of the "unseen observer" is useful, since most clients readily volunteer that previous journal writing has been addressed to "seen" audiences: e.g., "What would my lover think?" "What might people say?" "My mother might . . . ").

3. This is to not be viewed as a "writing experience," and therefore lists and sketchy observations may be the most useful. The skill of observing without instant analysis is essential.

The therapist's role in this stage is to elucidate the patterns of codependency rather than to give individuals specific suggestions or interpretations. The therapist minimizes his or her role of problem solver change-agent. While the therapist remains more of an observer of the client's process, he or she does not remain aloof. He or she connects with the clients via the pattern of codependency or specific content.

In Annon's model (1976) of sex therapy, giving permission to be a sexual being is the first and most important step in sex therapy. This model naturally lends itself well to the treatment of codependent clients. The model states that the therapist does not begin with methods of intensive therapy in which boundaries are invaded and interpretations given — and probing and confrontation are the rule. It is common to accept the client's statements and then give them permission to simply express feelings and views. The therapist also emphasizes that there are no "right" answers or "right" responses or other simple, magical answers to intimacy problems. Initially, we simply ask people to explore and to find out more about themselves and their responses. If clients are resistant to this approach, the resistance is accepted. Often we need to slow down the therapeutic process. These clients often deny their own complexity, as well as that of others, and they may never have paused to ask questions such as — "Who am I?" and "What do I want?" These basic questions are diverted because codependent clients are often compulsively engaged in "impression management" (Goffman, 1959) — devoting social energy to managing other's impressions of self. These clients want change in their intimate relationships without working on themselves. "Fix him or her" is the underlying message.

The opposite message is also heard often: "It's all my fault, and I don't know what I can do about it." A time limit is established so that the dependency on the therapy or therapist is not fostered. Instead of high levels of therapist intervention, there are high levels of information given.

STAGE TWO—
FOCUSING ON INTERACTION WITH OTHERS

The second stage of treatment helps clients focus on the "social me" or the "me in interaction." George Herbert Mead (1962) discusses a self that includes the subjective, spontaneous "I" and the social, role-fulfilling "me." In this stage, the treatment focuses on the interactional process of identity. Here the emphasis is on all the codependent client's relationships—past and present. All the authors ask each client to do an intensive investigation of his or her relationship history.

Relationships that the client considers significant are examined (past and present). Individual patterns or themes emerge. What is usually obvious is the tendency of each person to neglect or abuse himself or herself for the sake of relationships. Inevitably the resulting information is insightful, and out of this experience clients usually see some change in friendship dynamics, boundary limits, etc. Often the amount of identity one is receiving or demanding from other people's behavior (the symbiotic me) is surprising. The material used by each person is from their own self-observations logged in their journal.

Many of the authors' clients hold unhealthy attitudes toward intimacy. Common attitudes include:

— Intimacy doesn't exist.
— Intimacy will never be possible for me.
— Intimacy is something you take; it is never freely given.
— You can only be intimate if there is sex involved.
— Intimacy is power.
— Intimacy always makes you feel powerless.

In stage two, the goal is to encourage gentle self-confrontation. The client asks questions such as: "Who am I in relationships?", "What is me?", "What is not me?". As Erikson (1978) observed, engagement with others is the result and test of firm self-definition. Engagement, playing, and experimenting with relationship patterns is encouraged in order to begin the process of loosening old patterns.

The role of the therapist is to maintain the protective stance of stage one, while encouraging self-confrontation. During this stage, the boundaries between individual clients, the couple, or group members and the therapist begin to soften so that individuals can be joined and separated at the same or different times (Davis and Wallenbridge, 1981). To avoid the over-interpretation and boundary invasion by the therapist, it is helpful to avoid labeling client responses — even to oneself. Information about codependency is presented in generalities rather than in specific statements about the client's pattern. It is helpful to note, recognize, acknowledge and value each small change that occurs.

After a period of gentle confrontation, the therapist begins the process of firm confrontation with one's past and one's present. Through greater self impingement, rather than therapist impingement, the client identifies patterns and designs his or her own change strategies. Plans for change or self-launching are then started.

For example, one client wrote these self-launching plans for herself: (1) Genuine reinforcement for each step toward independence. (2) Continuous celebration for who I am and who I am becoming. (3) Believe in me and trust that I can take care of myself. (4) Permission to (a) screw up, (b) experiment, (c) change my mind, (d) live my life true to my type. Now the client is beginning to "be on his or her own side" as well as confront belief patterns and develop firm strategies for change. It is in this stage that clients are ready to say, "I . . . . "

In working with codependent clients who seem resistant to focusing on self, the authors strive to set a therapeutic environment that is time-limited and short-term — but that is still somewhat flexible and congruent with the natural learning time of each individual.

The assumptions of this model are that self-awareness or identity is fostered, at first, by information about codependent patterns rather than by personal feedback to the codependent client. The environment is structured so that everyone may just "be," and boundaries are preserved. Next, gentle confrontation is introduced that does not come from the therapist or others but from the codependent client. The environment is structured to facilitate this gentle self-confrontation by allowing for playfulness and experimentation.

STAGE THREE—
FOCUSING ON THE DYADIC RELATIONSHIP

Once the individuals in the relationship have begun resolution of stages one and two, they are ready to begin work as a couple in therapy. Specific methods of marital therapy can now be initiated. For example, improving dyadic communication is essential. Many lack basic communication skills. Communication skills can be taught through courses such as the Couples Communication Program developed at the University of Minnesota (Miller, Nunnally, & Wackman, 1979). Or, the therapist can utilize other models of teaching basic communication skills. In addition, the therapist can utilize the increasing use of the group treatment and aftercare couples groups found in many chemical dependency treatment centers.

Building trust in the relationship may be a challenging task, especially when trust has been so seriously destroyed by broken promises, denials, rationalizations, and false hopes. In more serious cases, verbal, physical, or sexual abuse leads to deep seated distrust, anger, and resentment. Trust is built on disclosure, honesty, and respect for individual boundaries. Trust is rebuilt when both partners are willing to focus on themselves and work on tasks in the first stages of treatment. If the first stages of treatment are successfully accomplished, trust is much less of an issue in this stage of intimacy building.

As part of intimacy building, a workshop focusing on their sexual attitudes and values is often recommended. A Sexual Attitude Reassessment (SAR) is recommended at a point in therapy when clients are ready to focus on the enrichment of their intimacy and sexual expression. SAR was originally developed to assist professionals reassess their sexual attitudes and values and to be more understanding of others. The authors have found this seminar helpful in the treatment of their clients. They have had the opportunity to adopt healthier attitudes that promote intimacy. In addition, SAR helps overcome feeling of shame about sexuality and improves communication about sexuality.

Ultimately, this stage of treatment helps the individuals in a dyadic relationship define themselves and their partners in a comfortable and balanced way so that they can relate without covert or overt codependency traits or states. It helps to remember that we know our separateness only so far as we live in connection to others. And, that we experience relationships only insofar as we differentiate others from the self.

CONCLUSION

Treatment of intimacy dysfunctions involves treatment of identity dysfunctions. This kind of treatment is a more pronounced issue when working with chemically dependent and codependent people. Treatment of these dyadic relationship patterns can be divided into three stages. Before direct treatment of the dyadic relationship begins, the therapist should be assured that the individuals in the relationship have begun resolution of the first two stages (either in their own development, through therapy, or both). This treatment approach does not require the total reworking of the client's total identity.

The goals are to facilitate reframing of one's past and present relationships in order to gain some personal power and to restore hope. Personal power and choice generates unity that is essential to a sense of identity. Hope comes when clients identify their painful dependencies as learned behaviors, feelings, and attitudes that can be unlearned. Treatment of codependency patterns helps clients believe that they have inner resources and that there are relationships that can affirm them. In cases where individuation or relating is seriously impaired (codependency state), long term individual treatment might be advised. However, for most chemically dependent and codependent relationships, the treatment model that has been described here is successful in treating intimacy and sexual difficulties for many individuals who possess varying degrees of codependency traits.

The essential point that therapists must recognize when attempting to perform this type of therapy approach is that the codependency traits in clients may take on various forms that include: (1) defiance, (2) hostility, (3) power plays, (4) idealized self-images, (5) compliance, (6) psychological withdrawal, (7) circumventive communication. As therapists, we should note how the client attempts to keep the focus on others (past or present).

The authors advise that the individual in the dyadic relationship first be given the opportunity to identify patterns as a spectator in a passive, non-personalized manner—whether in individual, couple, or group counseling. Gentleness coupled with increasing firmness is the ambience needed in order for clients to begin designing their own strategies for learning to meet their own dependency needs—and for launching themselves in autonomy. Success is neither guaranteed nor arrived at easily. Clients may not complete their journey toward self reliance in a relationship in a short time, but they may at least gain a good start, and they will often return later to deal with more complex problems as they develop more autonomy and more ability to engage in self-confrontation. The inside-out pattern has begun.

REFERENCES

Annon, J. S. (1976). The PLISSIT model: A proposed scheme for the behavioral treatment of sexual problems. *Journal of Sex Education and Therapy* Vol 2 (1): 1-15.
Cermak, T. L. (1986). Diagnostic criteria for codependency. *Journal of Psychoactive Drugs* Vol *18* (1): 15-20.
Coleman, E. (1987). Chemical dependence and intimacy dysfunction: Inextricably bound. *Journal of Chemical Dependency Treatment* Vol *1*.
Coleman, E. & Colgan, P. Boundary inadequacy in chemically dependent families. *Journal of Psychoactive Drugs* Vol *18* (1): 21-30.
Davis, M. & Wallbridge, D. (1981). *Boundary and Space: An Introduction to the Work of D. W. Winnicott.* New York: Brunner and Mazel.
Erikson, E. (Ed.) (1978). *Adulthood.* New York: Norton Press.
Gierymski, T. & Williams, T. Codependency. *Journal of Psychoactive Drugs* Vol *18* (1): 7-13.
Goffman, E. (1959). *The Preservation of Self in Everyday Life.* Garden City, NY: Doubleday.
Group for the Advancement of Psychiatry, Committee on the Family (1970). *The Field of Family Therapy* Vol *7*, Report No. 78.

Mead, G. H. (1962). Mind, self and society. In C. W. Morias (Ed.) *Mind, Self, and Society*. Chicago: University of Chicago Press, 135-226.

Mowrer, O. H. (1961). *The Crisis in Psychiatry and Religion*. New York: Van Nostrand.

Miller, S., Nunnally, E. & Wackman, D. (1979). *Talking Together* Minneapolis, MN: Interpersonal Communications Program, Inc.

Smalley, S. (1982). *Codependency: An introduction*. New Brighton, MN: SBS Publications.

Toward a Healthy Sexual Lifestyle Post Chemical Dependency Treatment

Sandra L. Nohre, MA

SUMMARY. Treatment of and recovery from chemical dependency surfaces numerous problems in relationships and sexual functioning. These problems will be discussed. The author believes that freedom from chemicals must be accompanied by the re-awakening of the physical senses and emotional responses. Sexual therapy can be an effective therapeutic approach. In reviewing the role of sexual therapy, this paper introduces a definition of sexuality. The journey toward a healthy sexual lifestyle for the chemically dependent person is an exploration through the areas of self-esteem, self-responsibility, communication, touching and intimacy. Awareness of one's personal values and attitudes are primarily essential to a healthy recovery.

The relationship between chemical dependency and family intimacy dysfunction has been well established (Coleman, 1982, 1987). The pain and stress of recovery as well as the common ensuing sexual problems inherent in the lives of these individuals has also been addressed frequently (Apter-Marsh, 1984). This paper explores areas of self-esteem, self-responsibility, communication, touching, and intimacy in the resolution of these problems and in the journey toward a healthy sexual lifestyle.

Sandra L. Nohre is a licensed psychologist and an ASSECT-certified sex therapist in private practice in Bloomington, MN and at the Program in Human Sexuality, Department of Family Practice and Community Health, Medical School, University of Minnesota, 2630 University Avenue S.E., Minneapolis, MN 55414.

© 1987 by The Haworth Press, Inc. All rights reserved.

DESCRIPTION OF THE PROBLEMS

For many people, the idea of rebuilding their sexual lives after treatment feels like an overwhelming task, not only personally but within their relationships as well. For some, it is often easier to avoid sex than to deal with the anxieties and fears that underlie healthy sexual functioning and intimacy. This method of coping can become a lonely experience. For others, delving into fears and anxieties regarding sexuality and intimacy is also a lonely process. Yet it has also been demonstrated that if sexual concerns are not dealt with during or following a treatment program, individuals are at a higher risk for recidivism. Returning to the chemicals of choice is a form of protection in order to avoid confronting the feelings related to chemical dependency, sexuality, and intimacy issues.

SEXUALITY ISSUES

The sexuality issues to be dealt with include fears, doubts, performance anxieties, sexual dysfunctions, sex roles, feelings of inadequacy and failure, and rejection. Whichever issues were present prior to the dependency are usually present following treatment. The difference is that issues post-treatment tend to be more powerful because the drugs are no longer present to alleviate the pain associated with anxieties and fears. Consequently, it is extremely important that chemically dependent individuals have a way of giving themselves permission to begin to confront the feelings, fears, anxieties and dysfunctions as these issues surface (Coleman, 1982).

The author believes that the fear of intimacy is synonymous with the fear of sexuality. This fear of intimacy is a major barrier towards the development of a healthy sexual lifestyle.

As we are learning more about the connections between chemical dependency and sexuality, it is also becoming clear that a good understanding of one's personal values and attitudes toward sexuality are primarily essential to a healthy recovery. These attitudes play a powerful role in how individuals respond to their life situations.

DEFINITION OF SEXUALITY

In order that there be a clear understanding of what is meant by sex and sexuality, the following definitions are being used for this paper.

The definition of sexuality: "Sexuality is that psychic energy which finds physical and emotional expression in the desire for contact, warmth, tenderness, and love." The author has added five components which encompass the definition of sexuality: physical, emotional, intellectual, spiritual, and social or interpersonal.

Physical

The body has the capacity for experiencing arousal, lubrication, orgasm, erection, and ejaculation. The capacity to enjoy the five physical senses varies with the body's sensual attunement. It is through the body that individuals express themselves sexually to the world around them. Consequently, body problems usually become sexual problems. Feeling positive toward one's body is an important step in feeling good about one's sexuality. Body image is often used as a validation of self. When one's body is liked and respected, it is easier to make sexual requests with a partner. Without body comfort, sexual expression is inhibited. Medications, drugs, alcohol, and over-indulgence in food affect libido, responsiveness, and sexual functioning.

Emotional

Sexual emotions need to be understood, identified, and expressed in order to experience the full range of sexual feelings, and to integrate emotions with thoughts. Denying or repressing feelings results in inhibited sexual responsiveness and can lead to aversiveness. In contrast, it can also be the precursor to acting out behaviors. Feeling positive emotionally enables giving self permission to be sexual in open and healthy ways.

Intellectual

The most powerful human "sex organ" is located in the mind. The mind has the ability to concentrate on sexual feelings and to affirm the body experiences. It also has the ability to allow sexual fantasy for arousal, or to repress fantasy and inhibit sexual arousal. Ultimately, the mind controls sexual response. Openness to sexual stimuli as well as the key to sexual arousal is a mental function. It also allows identification and clarification of sexual values and goals.

Spiritual

A key component in chemical dependency treatment and aftercare, as introduced through Alcoholics Anonymous, is the relationship between individuals and their Higher Power. This relationship can be viewed from several perspectives: the relationship to a Higher Power, to a God, to the individual's Higher Self. This component includes learning to trust the Higher Self, to discipline the self sexually, and to acknowledge desire as the desire for wholeness and health. Spirituality's the way to pattern or shape life-giving energies of the body, mind, and spirit. The sexual journey at its very core is a spiritual journey. Spirituality is necessarily inclusive of healthy sexuality. Spirituality demands reverence for self and others.

Interpersonal

Humans are created with a drive to be in relationships with others. In the unfearful state, humans search for connection and closeness, to be loved and to love. The search for connection and intimacy begins at birth, the process continues until death. Lacking this, the person feels alienated and alone. This social component is the culmination of the above four components as the search for meaningful relationships continues. Sex, as differentiated from sexuality, is defined as the behaviors in which people participate; as hugging, petting, oral sex, intercourse, self-pleasuring, etc. Human sexuality includes all that we are as human beings, from the beginning to the end of life. To be a person is to be sexual, whether there is genital sexual expression or whether celibacy or chastity have been chosen as a permanent or temporary lifestyle.

ROLE OF SEX THERAPY

Sex Therapy: Purpose

The chemically dependent person has learned to fear this natural process. To cope with fears and emotional pain, alcohol and drugs are used to inhibit the body's physical and emotional responses. With increasing inhibition of the physical senses, the range of sexual responsiveness becomes markedly narrowed. In order for the chemically dependent person to become sexually healthy again, the emotional responses as well as the physical senses need to be awakened and broadened.

Sex therapy can be very effective in this opening up process. A large proportion of the therapy takes place within the five physical senses: sight, sound, taste, touch, and smell. Whereas alcohol and drugs were used to release anxiety, sex therapists teach chemically dependent individuals breathing and relaxation techniques to help them cope more successfully with their anxieties and fears. Sex therapy can assist these persons by providing an opportunity to learn how to experience appropriate "highs" with themselves, by learning to relax and by becoming open to their own sexuality.

Sex Therapy: Education

Sex therapists also play an important educational role in the treatment of the problems associated with chemical dependency. It is important that clients are taught that sexuality is a natural, physiological process of the human body. Just as people are born with an appetite for food, so are they born with an appetite for sex. This appetite for sex can be suppressed and hidden by traumatic events, as well as by anger, depression, and dysfunctional relationships, but it can never be destroyed.

Masters & Johnson state that every 90 minutes during rapid eye movement (REM) sleep male infants erect and female infants lubricate. This life-long physiological process may be interrupted by disease, illness, or accident. Thore Langfeldt (1981) indicates that lubrication and erection begin prior to birth, during fetal development. Sexual functioning is the one physical process that need not be expressed, which makes possible the choice of short-term or long-term celibacy and chastity (Masters and Johnson, 1966 and 1974).

Human sexuality is more than just a biological phenomenon, however. The sociocultural and psychosexual components and their interactions also help shape self image and level of self esteem. These components have significant impact on relationships. Understanding sexuality thus becomes extremely complex. As a result, most persons experience their sexuality as a source of great pleasure as well as intense vulnerability. Because sexuality has the power to create such intense highs and lows, it can be a source of great fear.

STEPS TOWARD A HEALTHY SEXUAL LIFESTYLE

The journey from chemical dependency toward a healthy sexual lifestyle has many important steps. The author believes the following five components are key issues to be explored and resolved: self-esteem, self-responsibility, communication, touching, and intimacy.

Self-Esteem

The hallmark of a person who abuses chemicals is poor self-esteem. Turning to alcohol and drugs to cope with low self-esteem creates a dependency in which the ability to be intimate is virtually impossible except with the drug of choice. Looking to substitutes does not allow this self-worth to emerge or be maintained. These feelings of low self-esteem, doubts about self-worth and feelings of inadequacy make it difficult to develop a satisfying relationship. As the author's client, Nancy, said one day, "It is hard to be intimate when my level of self-esteem is so low." Building positive self-esteem is the bedrock of personal health, sexual health, and relationship health.

Self-Responsibility

Learning to take time to learn about self seems selfish to many people. Yet unless the individual learns to understand and know themselves, it is difficult to share and to give to others in a significant way. An ancient dictum strongly counsels, "Love your neighbor *as* yourself," not more than yourself, as most people learned. Taking time, "prime time," to understand self assumes the following: a high priority is given to working to understand and appreciate sensuality and to trust feelings once again; listening to the body and validating sexual needs and desires; accepting the body and its sexual arousal; understanding and appreciating the genitalia. Taking responsibility for one's orgasm through self-pleasuring versus partner sex can be an important way to experience sexual release when being in a sexual relationship could be potentially destructive to the recovery process. Some persons intentionally choose or are required by therapists to impose a temporarily celibate lifestyle while putting their lives in order.

Sexual self-responsibility, a concept that evolved during the 1970s, has helped to dispel some of the massive amounts of sexual mythology and misinformation that had been disseminated previously. Once seen as the sole responsibility of the male, sexual arousal and functioning have become a matter of individual determination and responsibility. Within a relationship, there is a fine line between self needs and partner needs. However, just as one person cannot assume responsibility for their partner's breathing, neither can they be responsible for another's sexual arousal, lubrication, erection, or orgasm. These can only be facilitated or enhanced with partner. An individual can choose to be responsive to their partner, but no one can control another person's physiological and emotional processes.

In learning about self-responsibility and appropriate boundaries, talking with other people or friends in a supportive, caring atmosphere can be an important avenue into self-understanding. Being assertive for oneself becomes easier with increased self-knowledge. Sexual self-responsibility and sexual assertiveness skills are necessary to help persons move out of passive roles, positions of powerlessness and a mind set that diminishes their sexual rights.

Communication

Meaningful communication presupposes two parts: (1) self-awareness; and (2) a willingness to share that self-awareness with another person (Miller, Nunnally, & Wackman, 1975).

Self-knowledge and awareness are generally required in order for persons to take sexual self-responsibility and to develop health relationships. Once developed, it is in the sharing of this knowledge that individuals become capable of a loving, caring, and intimate relationship. Likewise, effective sexual functioning happens when individuals know and understand themselves sexually (barring physical problems or diseases) and then become involved *with* each other rather than doing something *to* or *for* each other.

Satir (1972) states that "communication is an umbrella that covers and affects all that goes on between human beings. Communication is the greatest single factor affecting a person's health and his/her relationship to others." This includes sexual health.

Sexual problems in relationship are often due to a lack of communication. Even after learning positive communication skills, many couples express continued difficulty in communication of sexual issues. This is understandable given centuries in which sex was an unspeakable topic. Even today, when talking about sex is more acceptable, many can do so only through jokes or stories, rather than personal sharing. Since the area of sexuality is so vulnerable, talking seriously about sex creates insecurity and fear. Because of the fear of being hurt or rejected, many persons do not risk communicating their vulnerabilities, wants and needs sexually. What tends to occur is silence, evading, lying or "sexual games" which begin to permeate and distort the relationship.

However, when direct, honest communication with caring is practiced, very often the feelings of hurt or rejection can be de-emphasized. Couples in recovery must learn to deal with the feelings of anger and resentment in a direct and respectful way. This often means uncovering years of emotional pain.

It does take knowledge and practice in order to communicate and be intimate in a sexual relationship. Good communication skills are essential to creating solutions and developing the nature of the relationship in ways that are mutually satisfying. Recovering clients need opportunities to develop these skills. Though they may be skillful verbally in social situations, verbal intimacy skills may be a deficient area in their personal lives. It is rare to sustain intimacy over time without the intimacy of words as well. Learning to communicate skillfully and effectively forms the base and surrounds the whole field of sexual counseling and chemical dependency counseling.

Touching

Though verbal communication is very important for clarity and understanding interactions, words alone fail to convey the full meaning of intimacy. Persons long to communicate their deepest joys and fears, anxieties and love, and this longing achieves it's deepest significance through touch, a primal function.

By virtue of being human, all people need to touch and to be touched. Skin is the most fundamental sex organ. Montagu (1978) states: "The need for touch is a basic need that must be satisfied if the person is to survive." Infants need touch to survive physically and emotionally. Touch is a natural part of life in childhood. As we move toward adulthood, inhibitions repress the natural touching of childhood. We often observe individuals apologizing for even minimal, accidental touching.

One of the most misunderstood concepts in our society is the relationship of touching to sex. The implication that touching is a seductive or overt sexual act has caused many people to deny expression to their touching needs. They become unable to distinguish the need for and expression of sex from other feelings, equally intense. Hence, the confusing messages surrounding touching cause persons to question the motives and intentions of the toucher. An important task is to learn to differentiate between confusing, nurturing, sensual, sexual, and exploitative kinds of touch.

While chemically dependent persons are building intimacy

with their chemicals of choice, the desire and ability to be touched lessens. Physical contact may be limited to those moments when sexual contact is desired, often with one partner in the relationship feeling used and manipulated for sex. Touching then becomes a negative experience. Learning to touch in intimate ways can be a very threatening experience, especially if these persons are trying to relearn these skills following a breach of trust. Non-sexual touching (non-genital, non-erotic forms of touching) can enable individuals/couples to re-establish feelings of trust, loving and intimacy. Couples need to learn these tasks of giving and receiving touch to succeed in therapy and in their ongoing relationship.

Men and women tend to be conditioned differently in our society regarding touch. Women tend to separate more clearly their need for holding touch from sexual touch. Men often perceive touch as a prelude to intercourse or as an invitation to sex. Women will bargain with sex to get touching, whereas men tend to be more likely to bargain with touching to get sex. The battles that ensue are obvious (Hollender, 1970). In the 1980s, the sex of the bargainer may have changed and the sex roles may have become a little less distinct, but the dynamics continue in a similar fashion.

The difference between nurturing touch and sexual contact touch are lessons to be taught and learned throughout life. Otherwise, these individuals grow up exploiting others, being exploited, and are unable to make meaningful relationships in adulthood.

Over several years, the author has presented sexuality seminars in a prison setting. The majority of inmates, when asked about touch experiences in childhood, associated pain with touching and reported being touched (struck) only when they did something wrong. Only one-fifth of the men could recall any kind of nurturing touch in their families of origin. The lack of nurturing touch and the inability to learn nurturing touch gives important messages about the origins of violence (Prescott,1975). Bodies need nurturing touch to give a sense of wholeness and well-being to the self and in order to reciprocate nurturing touch.

Intimacy

Intimacy, generally defined, is expressions of caring and closeness without manipulation. The search for intimacy begins at birth and continues throughout life. During the life cycle, there are many different kinds of intimacy needs that must be met in order to develop a healthy sexual lifestyle.

Intimacy needs vary from the physical, emotional and spiritual to the recreational, intellectual, aesthetic, affectional, and social.

One client stated, "The two best ways I could kill pain was to get drunk or get laid. The loss of intimacy in my life created even greater pain." In recovery, the issues with intimacy that were present as the dependency developed will re-surface and be present after treatment. Recovering persons need permission to explore these feelings and fears, to share, to be accepting of themselves as sexual beings, to learn to touch again without old fears, to become affectional in new ways in their journey toward intimacy. The fear of intimacy is the major barrier in the recovery process (Mason, 1986).

When persons turn to alcohol or drugs in search of intimacy, a dependency is created which makes intimacy virtually impossible. In a therapy session one day, a recovering alcoholic husband in complete exasperation asked his wife why she wouldn't relax and have sex with him. In her frustration, she literally screamed at him, "How can you expect me to want to make love to you, when all you've been doing is making love to your bottle for 20 years." Later, in a calmer moment, she explained, "When he was making love to his bottle, there was no way I wanted to make love with him. And now that he's sober, I am still having difficulty letting go of those negative feelings. They remain strong and insistent despite the fact that I would like them to change." As professionals, it is necessary to realize that not only does the chemically dependent individual have a learned association between sex and chemicals, but so also does the co-dependent partner. Thus, the cycle broadens: more distance and alienation, less trust and intimacy, and lowered self-esteem.

Achieving intimacy is a multi-faceted task. Rebuilding the trust level may be extremely difficult. It implies being open and vulnerable, being willing to risk becoming emotionally available to partner once again, and being hurt—again. The critical issue becomes, "If I start to trust you, are you going to let me down again?" This can, in some instances, be a long and deeply frustrating process. One alcoholic husband during a therapy session said to his wife, "How long do I have to prove myself—prove that I can be trusted again?"

Though trust is not easily re-built, effective communication skills can begin to lay the foundation and hopefully accelerate the rebuilding process. Because the relationship between two persons can be mutually enhancing or destructive, the variable between those two elements lies in the commitment of the two individuals to work together to overcome negative sexual patterns that may have developed. Sexually, working together involves making a decision to become more intimate and to deal with unresolved issues.

Unacknowledged anger is a major inhibitor of sexual functioning and intimacy. Unexpressed anger blocks the normal flow of sexual feelings. Therapy cannot be effective because the resistance to change and the fear of being controlled are too high. Emotions can frustrate even the most skilled therapist utilizing the most current sexual knowledge and techniques. Learning to accept and then to express anger appropriately is a major factor in developing sexual intimacy.

INTIMACY AND TRUST

As people communicate and share ideas and feelings, trust begins to build. As trust builds, becoming vulnerable involves risk—risk of emotional pain, fear of failure and fear of success. It involves moving towards one another through a process of self-disclosure and other exploration. Self-disclosure may cause a person to feel so vulnerable that it forces them to withdraw from the relationship couple. The critical factor in healthy intimate relationships is being able to make choices: whether to move closer together or farther apart. Both require special and different kinds of strengths. The ability to risk being vulnerable means moving closer to create connections and to be able to survive rejection; choosing distance means a time for self-renewal, and the ability to experience wholeness without the partner. As risk-taking and sharing continue, the deeper is the intimacy that is created in the relationship.

INTIMACY AND SEX

A typical way to search for intimacy is through sex. Sex cannot create intimacy; in fact, sex can be an excellent way to avoid intimacy. If a couple is having sexual contact, listen carefully to their feeling descriptions following orgasm or intercourse. When the comments are, "I felt so lonely" or "I felt depressed afterwards," this is an indication that the intimacy level has not been achieved. Persons who seek orgasm as an end in itself are often left feeling lonely and deserted. Some couples even have an active sex life, but suffer from sensual deprivation and thus a lack of intimacy.

Finding intimacy in another person is also impossible, despite the fact that many chemically dependent persons try this method. Intimacy must first begin with the self. Learning to know and trust self are crucial steps to learning how to be intimate before intimacy is possible with another (Erikson, 1978). With chemical dependency, this level of self-awareness and self-esteem were shattered, if ever established. Each person in a relationship, therefore, must start on the road to self-awareness. Trust of self is a prerequisite to risk-taking in relationships.

CASE ILLUSTRATION

Karen came to the author seeking sex therapy six months after chemical dependency treatment, feeling ready to deal with her sexuality. Her husband of 15 years joined her for the session. "What I loved about alcohol was that it allowed me to let my child come out to play and now I can't play anymore. I'm serious all the time." As she cried, it was clear that this woman would have to learn to be playful once again or she would be at risk for recidivism. She continued that sex was always serious now and she could respond only rigidly. Intercourse had to occur in the "only acceptable, proper position—missionary." Foreplay and touch had become miserably uncomfortable and oral sex was re-pulsive. Yet, under the influence of alcohol, she allowed herself to experiment and to enjoy. Now sober, the pleasure was gone.

Getting high was Karen's way of dealing with inhibitions, guilt, and fear. Hence, she also had developed a learned association between the chemicals and her sexual behavior. Her task, as that of other chemically dependent persons who have learned to narrow their responses and close down their senses, is to open themselves up emotionally again to being fully alive sensually and then sexually.

Performance vs. Pleasure

Much of our society's emphasis is on performance. People and literature often put a major stress on productivity and sexual performance. Orgasm has become the measurement of sexual success or failure. Performance fears are paramount after treatment, such as worrying about erections, lubrication, ejaculation, orgasms, and enjoyment. Reducing performance pressure can be enhanced by utilizing the concept of pleasuring which involves the maximum development of the five physical senses and awareness of what is being experienced in the moment. Other awarenesses include communication, relaxation, massage, etc. It enables a person to be a more sensual being and then to express this sensuality in the context of a relationship. This can assist clients to experience receiving pleasurable highs through their own senses, rather than addictive chemical highs. Thus, when performance does not measure up to expectations, it need not be viewed as failure and become a wedge in the relationship. Rather, when the client experiences the sensual pleasure of each moment, erection or orgasm can take second place in the process. A deficient performance, instead of being devastating, can be accepted and even appreciated.

According to Ashley Montagu (1978), "The need for touching and body pleasure is the center of sexual activity. Sex without sensuality is a bore, whereas sensual intimacy usually is a good experience, regardless of orgasm or performance." If two partners are truly intimate, if they enjoy the special event of their being together and give themselves in total to sensuality and mutual pleasure, then climaxes can make no difference—no wedges.

CONCLUSION

Sexuality is extremely complex. It involves the physical, intellectual, emotional, spiritual, and social self. It is an integral and valuable part of self. It can be ignored or honored. It can be acted out or acted upon. It can be healthy or dysfunctional. Our clients can choose to ignore their sexuality and pretend it doesn't exist, or they can choose to honor their sexuality with awareness and joy.

A basic assumption is that professionals undertaking this journey with their clients are first of all personally comfortable with their own sexuality, and professionally comfortable dealing with sex-related topics. It is assumed they have accurate and current information regarding these topics. The professional's own attitudes, anxieties and/or comfort directly affect the client through verbal as well as non-verbal messages. Genuineness, warmth, and empathy are personal qualities that enhance the permission-giving process so that clients can relieve guilt and shame and begin to deal effectively with intimacy issues. It is imperative that sexual health professionals know their own vulnerabilities and possess strong ethical boundaries so that the clients are not exploited and minimal negative transference occurs.

Assisting the chemically dependent and co-dependent persons on this journey back to the sensual self and to the discovery of intimacy must be done with integrity and respect.

REFERENCES

Apter-Marsh, M. The Sexual Behavior of Alcoholic Women While Drinking and During Sobriety. *Alcoholism Treatment Quarterly. 1* (3), 35-48.
Coleman, E. 1982. How Chemical Dependency Harms Marital and Sexual Relationships. *Medical Aspects of Human Sexuality. 16*, 42n-42cc.
Coleman, E. 1982. Family Intimacy and Chemical Abuse: The Connection. *Journal of Psychoactive Drugs. 14*, 153-158.
Coleman, E. 1983. Sexuality and the Alcoholic Family: Effects of Chemical Dependence and Co-Dependence Upon Individual Family Members. In Golding, P. (Ed.) *Alcoholism: Analysis of a World-Wide Problem*. Lancaster, England: MIP Press Limited.

Coleman, E. & Schaefer, S. 1986. Boundaries of Sex and Intimacy Between Client and Counselor. *Journal of Counseling and Development. 64,* 341-344.
Erickson, E.H. 1978. *Adulthood.* New York: Norton Press.
Hollender, M. 1970. The Need or Wish to Be Held. *Archives of General Psychiatry.* May, 64-74.
Langfeldt, T. Child Sexuality: Development and Problems. *Childhood & Sexuality: Proceedings of International Symposium.* Samson, Jan-Marc (Ed.), Montreal: Editiones Etudes, Vivantes.
Langfeldt, T. Sexual Development in Children. *Adult Sexual Interest in Children.* Editors: Cook, M. & Howells, K. London: Academic Press.
Langfeldt, T. 1981. Processes in Sexual Development. *Children & Sex: New Findings New Perspectives.* Editors: Constantine, L., Martinson, F.
Lidell, L. 1984. *The Book of Massage.* New York: Simon & Shuster.
Mason, M. March, 1986. *Intimacy.* Center City, MN: Hazelden Press.
Mason, M. Sexuality and Fear of Intimacy as Barriers for Recovery for Drug Dependent Women. Editors: Reed, B., Beshner, C. & Mondanara, J. *Treatment Services for Drug Dependent Women. II,* Washington, D.C. US Government Printing Office, for US Department of Health and Human Services.
Masters, W. and Johnson, V. 1966. *Human Sexual Response.* Boston: Little, Brown and Company.
Masters, W. and Johnson, V. 1974. *The Pleasure Bond.* Boston: Little, Brown and Company.
Miller, S., Nunnally, E. and Wackman, D. 1975. *Alive and Aware.* Minneapolis: Printing Arts, Inc.
Montagu, A. 1978. *Touching, The Human Significance of Skin.* New York: Harper & Row Publishers.
Powell, D., Ed. 1984. *Alcoholism & Sexual Dysfunction: Issues in Clinical Management.* New York: The Haworth Press.
Prescott, James. 1975. Body Pleasure and the Origins of Violence. *Futurist.* April, pp 64-74.
Satir, V. 1972. *Peoplemaking.* Palo Alto, CA: Science and Behavior Books, Inc.

Intimacy, Aging and Chemical Dependency

John Brantner, PhD

Intimacy means many things to different people, but there is little to be gained by being fussy, legalistic or too particular in definition. Intimacy embraces much and implies more. We call intimate that relationship which, with a satisfactory degree of mutuality, includes most of these eight qualities or characteristics. It need not include them all.

1. It seems for most to require something like *"equality"* in *status*, power, and vulnerability. Therefore, intimacy does not easily exist between employer and employee, between parent and child, between teacher and student, between warden and prisoner, between officer and enlisted rank, or in other relationships of large inequality.
2. Intimacy is found in a relationship of *love*. Love is wider and broader than intimacy but intimacy seems to be based on love. However, it should be noted that love need not, and usually in its higher, more developed levels, does not include intimacy. Love comes in many varieties, for example; Eros, Philia, Fraternity, Patria, Agape.
3. Intimacy is found in a relationship of *affection* — of mutual positive regard and reciprocated delight.
4. It is found in a relationship of *closeness*, nearness, and proximity — both emotional and physical. At times it is mea-

---

The late Dr. Brantner was Professor of Psychiatry, Medical School, University of Minnesota.
Requests for reprints may be sent to Eli Coleman, Program in Human Sexuality, 2630 University Avenue S.E., Minneapolis, MN 55414.

© 1987 by The Haworth Press, Inc. All rights reserved.

sured in centimeters; it nearly always has an outer limit in kilometers. It is very difficult to initiate, or even to maintain an intimate relationship if one of the pair is in Chicago and the other in Budapest.
5. Intimacy is found in a relationship of *vulnerability* and openness, the obverse and reverse of the same coin. In these relationships it is easy to wound or to be wounded. We are tender in both meanings of that word: our own sore spots are revealed, and we are solicitous of the sensitivities of the other.
6. It is found in a relationship of *understanding*, acceptance and patience. The old-fashioned word is "long-suffering."
7. For many it is almost necessarily found in a relationship of *loyalty* and its counterpart *exclusivity*.
8. It is found in a relationship that is open to all the richness and varieties of expressions of *sexuality*.

Intimate relationships are not absolutely necessary for survival. They are necessary for reasonably good mental health and for reasonably good social health. Some achieve it gloriously, early in life; they develop and grow in the relationship, enriching and increasing one another, until the death of one partner finds the other completed, made whole, never needing to know it further, never seeking it again. As widowed persons they seem to maintain a kind of intimacy and loyalty that reaches beyond or survives the death of the partner. They are also able to enter into a variety of supportive and compensating relationships.

Some, sadly and for a variety of reasons, are incapable of intimacy. This is most poignant when the incapacity is acknowledged by the person. An anonymous author a few years ago, suggesting that children should have the opportunity at age 14 to choose a new family recognized that his own childhood experience made intimacy nearly impossible for him. He said, "I am not unaware that . . . I am a very cold-hearted man. I might have done better transferred [as a child] to a new family, not just by receiving love, but through learning to give it—a lack I mourn as much or more than my failure to receive it" (1974). For most it is, throughout the life cycle a *desideratum*. They want it, they need it, they see it as the potentially achievable ideal. They suffer in its accurately perceived absence.

INTIMACY AND AGING

In this, what is the effect of aging? As always there are two contributions of aging: the effect of chronological age — the passage of years, and the effects of cohort — the effect of a particular history. "How old are you?" and "When were you born?" are two significantly different questions.

HOW OLD ARE YOU? There are three major effects of the passage of years:

1. There is continual attrition of the community of social relationships. With the passage of time we experience departures and deaths at all levels of sociability. We have fewer casual encounters with other people, we have fewer acquaintances. We lose friends and lovers. With age, both our kin and our kith decrease in numbers. The death of the accustomed intimate lover is especially difficult to bear.
2. Older people must deal with the learned, socially conditioned denigration and devaluing of the self, especially the sexual self. Our society in both direct and subtle ways teaches us that youth is comely and attractive; age is ugly and unattractive. "Old is ugly; I am old, therefore — ."
3. There are, of course, the very real biological shifts and changes. These are modifiable, compensable, capable of rehabilitation. Nonetheless, in all functions which we know how to measure, there is a gradual, threefold decline. This applies to all animal life. It is true of giraffes, and for all I know, spiders and moths. In the first, none of us jump as high, run as well, calculate, associate, or solve problems with the nimbleness and coordination we showed earlier. Secondly, we do not lift as heavy of weights nor push as strongly as we did before; there is a gradual, sometimes reversible loss in force. Third, touching all functions, whatever we do we do less quickly in our later years. The biological shifts and changes are mostly declines in agility,

strength, and speed. These combine to hamper the search in later years, leading us to devalue our performance in all the intimate skills.

WHEN WERE YOU BORN? The effects of cohort membership are strong, especially in a revolutionary era. Individuals born before World War I know most poignantly the effects of changing social expectations and possibilities. These effects may be transitional and apply only to the present cohorts of aging people. Change affects the future but operates in the context of past expectations and socializations. As the assistant demon said to Satan on his throne in Hell about ten or fifteen years ago, "What are we going to do with all those Catholics that ate meat on Fridays?" People born before World War I have seen marked changes in marriage rates, and in the frequency and acceptability of divorce. They have seen certain sexual behaviors, whether performed cross- or same-sex change from savagely punished felonies to tolerated and accepted behaviors. They must deal now with the scary possibilities of sexual intimacy without marriage, of extramarital affairs. They must deal with the recognition of continued sexual need throughout the life span and the possibility of alternative, non-genital, sexual expression. They must now consider cross-generational sexual possibilities and the possibility of same-sex intimacy. They were taught to disapprove of masturbation and reject it; now they must come to see it as a neutral or even positive experience. Of course in history and life experiences within any cohort there are great individual differences. Within a cohort, sexual adjustment ranges from celibacy to full and uninhibited sexuality. One might find in those born around 1895 prim and virginal individuals as well as lusty cavorters.

In the last quarter or third of the life span intimacy interacting with aging presents us with a situation of complexity, of uncertainty and change. For many this is a situation of regret, of sadness, and a clearly perceived lack or need. This lack or need will be differently expressed, possibly denied. Persons working with the aging population must have great sensitivity and skill in diagnosis and assessment of these issues.

INTIMACY AND ALCOHOL

What is the impact of alcohol and alcohol dependence? (Of course, this includes other anesthetic or consciousness-altering drugs or medications.)
Sentimentality is often mistaken for and substituted in place of genuine emotional response. Sentimentality is easily, readily and quickly accessible, non-demanding, and generally pandered to in our society. *Intimacy* like all great mature and developed emotional responses (e.g., devotion to country, love, developed religious faith, commitment to service) is difficult, demanding, and probably not accessible to all, and requiring a lifelong struggle. *Alcohol intensifies sentimentality*; it offers the conviction that one is making a mature and fulfilling emotional response when one does nothing of the sort. It provides a comfortable illusion of intimacy in life and relationships. One weeps at films and novels; feels warm and cozy at the sight of young lovers. One lies on the narrow cot drunkenly transported to a crowded bed.

Intimacy always challenges us, love makes demands, and friendship obliges. *Alcohol excuses us from obligation.* Drunk we need not accommodate another's needs, consider another's longings, or change our own set and self-centered ways.

Shyness, self-doubt, uncertainty, and a fear of rebuff retard or restrain many in the development of relationships, especially of intimate ones. *Alcohol dissolves shyness.* The tentative and shy entertain drunken dreams of boldness and adventure. If they act on them then, they only demonstrate their hopeless ineptitude and experience the added distress of self-loathing the next morning.

Loneliness makes many uncomfortable, dissatisfied, and sad who have not learned the techniques for adding new acquaintances, replenishing friendship, finding love and intimacy. This is especially sad for many of the elderly, undersocialized by attrition and loss. *Alcohol famously assuages loneliness.*

Alcohol is thus multiply attractive and a false friend. It is like pneumonia, another false friend of the aging population. It offers a totally unsatisfactory solution which at the same time makes all other solutions impossible.

TREATMENT

In addition, the lack of intimacy may be only one of the many causal and contributing factors in alcoholism in the aging population. The treatment of alcoholism at any age requires attention to each of its many causes. Neglect of any one is likely to lead to unsatisfactory treatment and relapse. There are many programs for the treatment of alcoholism in this population. No matter which route is followed some attention should be paid to possible problems of intimacy. With regard to treatment and intervention in problems of intimacy and alcoholism in the later years (or for any age), a few practical suggestions can be offered.

1. As always we should start with a sort of retreat, especially from current, tension-filled relationships, a temporary drawing back from the search for intimacy, a withdrawal from the fray. We should be able to say to the anguished one, "Cool it for now." As is often said in the various 12-Step programs, "Easy does it." This is exactly comparable to the temporary separation often advised in tense but solvable marital difficulty.
2. A thorough re-assessment of self and of personal, social, and sexual needs is necessary. The goal here is to recognize and accept and affirm oneself as real, valid, imperfect, and incomplete. As Alex Stevens, the poet, said at 80, "I am content to be what I am not content to stay" (1980). In this phase special efforts may be bent at building self-esteem and possibly changing lifestyle. It is possible to explore some changes in costume, carriage, manner, appearance, and style which may convince people that they may be more attractive to others than they thought.
3. One should start with redefinition of expectations and demands made on others. We must see that it is not reasonable, wise, or safe to demand or expect another to meet our deepest needs. As Henri Nouwen (1979) said:

> When we expect a friend or lover to be able to take away our deepest pain, we expect from him or her something that cannot be given by human beings. No human being can understand us fully, no human being can give us un-

conditioned love, no human being can offer constant affection, no human being can enter into the core of our being and heal our deepest brokenness. When we forget that and expect from others more than they can give, we will be quickly disillusioned; for when we do not receive what we expect, we easily become resentful, bitter, revengeful, and even violent. (p.41)

4. To come to see, and accept, and affirm others as real, valid, imperfect, and incomplete. This is both disappointing and yet liberating and exciting.
5. Perhaps to try again to enter into a relationship of intimacy, combining sex and love, but now recognizing that that relationship is basically nearly impossible — a relationship between two highly self-respecting individuals who somehow forget about themselves in a relationship which is at once delicate and strong, fragile and robust, risky and safe. Perhaps now we can entertain an oddly re-defined demand, saying to the other, "I will demand of your time, your interest, and your body only what you freely offer."
6. Perhaps, on the other hand, we may now decide honorably and knowingly that we can postpone the search for an intimate relationship. Postponement reduces both the pressure and the anguish. It gives us time to explore and practice the art of intimacy with self, with friends, with supportive others in the various treatment programs. When our gains in recovery are consolidated then we can move again into an intimate relationship of commitment, intensity, and sex; this time sure, strong, and sober.

Perhaps in all this we may be able to find in the last third or quarter of the life span that our cohort-based inhibitions can be transformed into liberation. Perhaps we can decide that the chronological age-based changes are never improved by the false friend alcohol which further reduces coordination, speed, and strength. We may also discover that all our functions can be improved by sober and wholesome use and exercise. Perhaps we can discover — again for some, freshly for others — the possibility of intimate relationships, mutually rewarding and mutually satisfying. Perhaps then we will watch the whole matter recede from a pain-filled and anguished center to a delightful and joyous periphery where it probably belongs.

REFERENCES

Anonymous (1974). Confessions of an Erstwhile Child. *The New Republic.* June 15, 1974, pp. 11-13.
Nouwen, Henri J.M. (1979). *Clowning in Rome.* Garden City: Image Books, Doubleday and Company.
Stevens, Alex (1980). An 80-years Self-Portrait. *The New Yorker.* April 7, 1980, p. 119.